# ATTENTION DEFICIT DISORDER

Professor Ashoka Jahnavi Prasad

Copyright © 2017 by Professor Ashoka Jahnavi Prasad

All Rights Reserved

This book contains material protected under International and Federal Copyright Laws and Treaties.

Created in Switzerland

This work is dedicated to mt teacher Sula Wollf,one of the pioneers of Child Psychiatry

## Table of Contents

Authors' Note

Introduction: Are "Alternative Treatments" Good Alternatives?

SECTION I: Attention Deficit Hyperactivity Disorder and Learning Disabilities: An Overview

    Chapter 1 What Is Attention Deficit Hyperactivity Disorder?

    Chapter 2 What Are Learning Disabilities?

SECTION II: Effective Treatments for ADHD and Learning Disabilities

    Chapter 3 How New Treatments Are Evaluated: Science, Pseudoscience, and Quackery

    Chapter 4 Effective Treatments for ADHD

    Chapter 5 Effective Treatments for Learning Disabilities

SECTION III: Out of the Mainstream: Controversial Treatments for Learning and Attention Problems

    Chapter 6 Pills and Potions

    Chapter 7 Dietary Interventions

    Chapter 8 Training Approaches to Treatment

    Chapter 9 Miscellaneous Approaches

Concluding Remarks: Where Do We Go from Here?

References

Addenda

## Authors' Note

The American Psychiatric Association has officially adopted the term "Attention Deficit Hyperactivity Disorder" (ADHD) to describe the condition commonly referred to as "Hyperactivity" or "Attention Deficit Disorder." Although Attention Deficit Hyperactivity Disorder may most accurately describe the condition, it can be unwieldy; so we often use the more common terms, interchangeably, throughout this book.

For convenience, we use the masculine "he" to indicate both genders.

# Introduction
## Are "Alternative Treatments" Good Alternatives?

The most conservative estimates suggest that at least 3 to 5 percent of all children have Attention Deficit Hyperactivity Disorder (ADHD), a condition the American Psychiatric Association includes among the so-called "disruptive behavior disorders." These disorders are characterized by behavior that is disruptive and disturbing to others in the child's environment. In comparison with children of similar age, children with ADHD have difficulty maintaining attention and remaining on-task, especially if the task is somewhat routine or monotonous. Children with ADHD are also quite impulsive, often acting before they think about the likely consequences of their actions. In addition, many ADHD children are much more fidgety, restless, and active than their age-mates, especially in situations which call for quiet or subdued behavior.

Children with ADHD often have other problems, including learning difficulties and poor school performance. As many as one quarter actually have documented *learning disabilities*; that is, there is a significant discrepancy between their overall intellectual abilities and their ability to learn academic skills. Despite an apparently normal or even superior capacity to learn, learning-disabled children lag far behind their classmates in their struggle to master reading, spelling, writing, and other academic tasks.

Just as many ADHD children suffer from learning disabilities, the converse is true, as well: of the 5 to 10 percent of children in the United States who are learning- disabled, about one third also have ADHD. From these figures, we can conclude that between 5 and 10 million children in the United States have ADHD and/or learning disabilities.

In centuries past, these children were capable of blending into a work force primarily driven by manual labor. Many were simply released from school and written off as bad, or stupid, or lazy. Some were warehoused in special education programs or juvenile detention facilities; others were sent off to boarding school or to join the army; still others simply drifted into low-paying jobs and a marginal existence on the fringes of society. Although some exceptional individuals like Winston Churchill, who had ADHD, and Thomas Edison, who was learning-disabled, overcame their early difficulties and went on to achieve great personal and professional success, many more did not.

It is to the credit of our society—and thanks to the unstinting efforts of thousands of dedicated parents and professionals—that we no longer tolerate such conditions for these children. In the late 1970s, largely through the efforts of parent-professional support groups like the Association for Children and Adults with Learning Disabilities, Public Law 94-142, the Education for All Handicapped Children Act, was enacted. This law, reauthorized in 1990 as the Individuals with Disabilities Education Act, mandates appropriate educational services for children with learning disabilities and other handicapping conditions, in every state in the country. Similar laws have since been enacted in other countries, including Canada.

More recently, there has been a tremendous upsurge of interest in the problems of children with ADHD. This interest is reflected not only in the increased number of books and articles in the scientific literature but also in the explosion of material directed at parents and teachers. Parents and professionals have joined forces in support groups, such as the Attention-Deficit Disorder Association (ADDA) and the Attention Deficit Disorder Advocacy Group (ADDAG), which have sprung up across the country. The largest of these is Children and Adults with Attention Deficit Disorders (CH.A.D.D.). Founded in 1987, this organization currently has chapters in all fifty states and a membership in excess of twenty thousand. Parent-professional groups such as CH.A.D.D. play a major role in drawing attention to the special needs of ADHD children and in lobbying to see that these needs are met. Thanks to their efforts, for example, the United States Department of Education issued a policy statement in September 1991 in which children with ADHD were expressly recognized as eligible for special education and related services under federal law. This represents a major victory for ADHD children, many of whom were formerly denied special services in school systems in which ADHD was not recognized as a handicapping condition.

**MYTHS, MISINFORMATION, AND THE MEDIA**

The problems of children with ADHD have also attracted the attention of the media. In fact, if television and the popular press are any indication, ADHD is the "in" childhood disorder of the 1990s. With a great deal of heat but very little light or enlightenment, this condition has been showcased on a host of radio and television talk shows. It has also been featured in popular magazines, newspaper columns—even in the tabloids we read while standing in the checkout lane at the supermarket.

Although this publicity has led to increased public awareness about ADHD, it has also led to a proliferation of myths and misinformation about the disorder and the methods used to treat it. The end result, in many ways, has been more confusion than clarification. All too often, parents are among those who are most confused, and parents can be easy prey indeed when faced with programs which are touted as helpful to their children.

As we will discuss, there are proven treatments for children with ADHD and learning disabilities (LD). But let's be very clear: when we use the term "proven," we refer only to those treatments which have met rigorous scientific tests of their effectiveness. Testimonials from satisfied customers are not enough, nor are celebrity endorsements or other forms of media hyperbole. To merit the term "proven," a treatment must meet very strict standards.

To repeat: there are treatments which have been shown to help many children with ADHD and learning disabilities. Unfortunately, these well-established treatments are not the stuff of which headlines are made. Instead, journalists and television reporters have gravitated toward new and unusual treatment programs which offer the promise of a miracle cure. A few of these "alternative treatments" may ultimately stand up to close scientific scrutiny. Some, however, represent little more than wishful thinking, while others are actually the work of charlatans and quacks whose principal interest is in lining their own pockets.

**BUYER BEWARE!**

Raising children is a demanding job under the best of circumstances. How much more difficult the task becomes for the parent of a child who suffers from ADHD or learning disabilities—or both. Since daily life with these children is often so full of confusion, frustration, and heartache, it is understandable that parents can become desperate in their search for answers. It is also understandable that, in their desperation, they welcome any new treatments which offer hope for their children. Thus, they may turn to treatments which claim to provide solutions but which have not really been shown to be effective, at least according to the standards by which the scientific community judges effectiveness.

This is a very real danger! No matter how intelligent or well educated parents might be, few have the training or the expertise to evaluate the effectiveness of new treatments which promise to help children with ADHD or learning disabilities. To begin with, simply locating the relevant information can be a formidable task. Where, for example, does one go to find the journal *Acta Psychiatrica Scandinavica*? Then, of course, there is the task of translating scientific jargon into some semblance of English: what does "focal cerebral hypoperfusion" mean? Scientific prose does not make for easy reading. Finally, evaluating the research methods and techniques used and then comparing the results of different studies can be formidable tasks, even for a trained professional.

**USING THIS BOOK**

To help parents, educators, and health-care professionals find a way through this maze, we have written this book. In it, we summarize what is currently known about the causes, the assessment, and the treatment of ADHD and learning disabilities.

Specifically, in Section I we explain the way in which ADHD and learning disabilities are diagnosed and evaluated, and we review what is known about the causes of these disorders. We also pay special attention to many of the popular myths and misconceptions which have led to so much confusion about these conditions.

In Section II, we describe the methods used by the scientific community to evaluate new treatment methods for ADHD and learning disabilities, and we compare this approach with the way in which some "alternative treatments" come to public attention. Using this analysis as a guideline, we then provide an overview of those treatment approaches which have well-established track records for success.

Section III provides an overview of controversial treatments which have been put forth as helpful to children with ADHD and learning disabilities. For each of these alternative treatments, a summary and evaluation of the scientific evidence is provided so that you, the reader, can make well-informed decisions concerning the treatment approaches most likely to help the child or children with whose special needs you are concerned.

# SECTION I
## Attention Deficit Hyperactivity Disorder and Learning Disabilities: An Overview

# Chapter 1

## What Is Attention Deficit Hyperactivity Disorder?

Over the course of this century, a bewildering variety of terms have been used to describe the condition we now call "Attention Deficit Hyperactivity Disorder" (ADHD). These terms include "minimal brain damage" (or "dysfunction"), "hyperkinesis," "hyperactivity," and "attention deficit disorder." Although the label has changed many times, the problem itself has remained constant over the years.

### WHO IS THE ADHD CHILD?

How do you recognize a child who has ADHD? He is the child who:

- Is indistinguishable from other children on the playground but who sticks out like the proverbial sore thumb in school, church, and other settings in which he must sit quietly and pay attention.

- Is obviously bright and creative but has difficulty learning in the classroom because he never finishes his work, loses books and papers, and can't get organized to plan, begin, or follow through on a task.

- Needs to have instructions repeated several times and, even then, has difficulty following them.

- Can sit for hours with an activity of his choice but has difficulty sticking with chores or schoolwork for more than a few minutes.

- Has a sweet and caring nature but blows up over small issues and creates crises over minor mishaps.

- Wants very much to please but is never quite able to live up to the expectations of those around him.

Of course, children are more active than adults. In fact, when parents of five-year-old boys are queried, as many as half describe their children as excessively active. And like the rest of us, children have days when they are disorganized and absentminded or days when they are irritable and easily frustrated.

Since the problems of the ADHD child are exaggerated forms of problems common to all children, how do you know when "too much is too much"? How do you decide whether your bouncy, active youngster is simply "all boy" or whether his high energy signals a problem? If he daydreams in class, does he have attentional problems or is he just bored? If he responds to his sister's taunts by thumping her a good one, is he too explosive or is this just normal sibling rivalry?

The American Psychiatric Association offers guidelines to be used by professionals as part of the diagnostic process for Attention Deficit Hyperactivity Disorder. These guidelines should never be used in isolation and they are far from perfect. However, they are helpful because they provide a common language and a set of common standards by which professionals can make a diagnosis.

The guidelines, outlined in the *Diagnostic and Statistical Manual of Mental Disorders,* (third Edition, revised, 1987),[1] are as follows.*

A. A disturbance of six months or more, during which at least eight of the following behaviors are present. The child:

  1. Often fidgets with hands or feet or squirms in seat (in adolescents, may be limited to subjective feelings of restlessness).

  2. Has difficulty remaining seated when required to.

  3. Is easily distracted by extraneous stimuli.

  4. Has difficulty awaiting turn in games or group situations.

  5. Often blurts out answers to questions before they have been completed.

6. Has difficulty following through on instructions from others (not due to oppositional behavior or failure to understand the directions); for example, fails to finish chores.

7. Has difficulty sustaining attention in tasks or play activities.

8. Often shifts from one uncompleted activity to another.

9. Has difficulty playing quietly.

10. Often talks excessively.

11. Often interrupts or intrudes on others; for example, butts into other children's games.

12. Often doesn't seem to listen to what is being said.

13. Often loses things necessary for tasks or activities at school or at home (for example, toys, pencils, books, assignments).

14. Often engages in physically dangerous activities without considering possible consequences (not for the purpose of thrill seeking); for example, runs into street without looking.

B. Onset of these problems occurs before the age of seven.

## CORE PROBLEMS

If you read this list carefully, you will see that these apparently diverse problems can be grouped into three categories:

· Attentional problems

· Difficulty controlling impulsive responding

· Excessive motor activity

Although these problems do not always occur together (some children have problems only with attention, for example), a majority of children who are diagnosed with ADHD have problems in all three areas. Let's examine each area more closely, discussing myths and misunderstandings as we go along.

*Attention*

In comparison with others his age, the ADHD child has difficulty concentrating and paying attention. His problems are particularly pronounced when he is faced with routine, monotonous activities. Under these circumstances, he is more easily distracted than his age-mates.

*Table 1: Myths and Facts about ADHD*

| Myth | Fact |
| --- | --- |
| A child doesn't have ADHD if he can pay attention to TV or other activities which interest him. | A child with ADHD has difficulty sustaining attention when an effort is required to do so. |
| All children with ADHD are excessively active. | Children need not be hyperactive to merit a diagnosis of ADHD. |
| Most ADHD children become delinquents. | ADHD and Conduct Disorder are separate disorders with different causes and outcomes. |
| The ADHD child's problems reflect poor parenting and/or a dysfunctional family. | Parents are not to blame for the primary problems of ADHD. |
| Food allergies and poor diet are the primary causes of ADHD. | The relationship between diet and ADHD has not been consistently demonstrated. |

Teachers describe such a youngster as a daydreamer. They complain that he is often off-task, engaging in a host of activities other than the one the teacher has assigned. In the home, parents describe a child who takes forever to do chores and can't be counted on to complete even the simplest tasks. For example, if the family pet really had to depend on him for nourishment, it would soon starve. At meals, this child is always the last to finish. Sent upstairs to dress for school, he can be found scant minutes before the bus arrives wearing only underpants and playing with the gerbil.

On the other hand, when this youngster is engaged in an activity of his choosing—be it Nintendo, dress-up, Legos, baseball cards, or just annoying his sibling—a combination of a crowbar and dynamite isn't enough to turn his attention to other matters. This, then, gives rise to the first of many myths about children with ADHD.

**Myth A Child Doesn't Have ADHD if He Can Pay Attention to TV or Other Activities Which**

**Interest Him.**

**Fact A Child with ADHD Has Difficulty Sustaining Attention When an Effort Is Required to Do So.**

Like the other core symptoms of ADHD, attentional problems fluctuate, depending on the situation. ADHD children have been described as having an "attentional bias toward novelty" because they seem to need more stimulation and variety than other children. Their attentional problems are much more pronounced in familiar or boring situations. Rote tasks, which require much repetition (like many school assignments), are torture for them.

On the other hand, these same children may have no apparent difficulty maintaining attention in other situations, especially those which are stimulating and interesting to them. It is important to note, however, that television producers and video game companies spend huge sums of money to produce programs and games which will hold the viewer's attention with little or no effort required on his part. (Isn't it interesting to speculate about what might happen if these resources were spent on developing academic programs and materials?)

Another factor affecting the ADHD child's ability to concentrate is time of day: his performance in the morning is generally better than it is in the afternoon and evening. The ADHD child is also better able to focus his attention when he has the undivided attention of an adult, than when he must work independently or share attention with others in a group.

Because the ADHD child's ability to pay attention varies so much with different situations, an observer is likely to conclude that the child is simply lazy and could concentrate quite well "if he really wanted to." This means that a child with ADHD is doubly penalized for his attentional deficits: not only is it more difficult than his parents and teachers realize for him to concentrate and complete tasks, but if he slacks off, he is chastised for laziness and lack of motivation.

*Impulsivity*

The ADHD child has a tendency to fling himself headlong into life, acting first and thinking about it later— if at all. His style is such that his motto might well be "Ready! Fire! ... Oops! ... Aim!" In fact, the inability of the ADHD child to inhibit impulsive behavior is so pronounced that many experts in the field now consider this problem, rather than attentional difficulties, to be the hallmark of ADHD.

Parents and teachers will recognize this youngster as the one who constantly calls out in class, interrupts the conversation of others, and plunges into a task or activity before he has listened to the directions. Because he does not take the time to plan ahead, his work is done in a disorganized, haphazard fashion. Chores and school assignments are often completed in a rush and are marred by careless errors. Peers find him annoying because he must always be first in line and can't wait for his turn in games.

Children with ADHD have great difficulty following rules. They are also "repeat offenders" who do not seem to learn from experience, no matter how many times they are punished for the same infraction. It's not that they don't know or understand the rules—indeed, they can recite chapter and verse. Rather, the problem lies in their inability to think before they act.

Another appropriate slogan for the ADHD child might be "I want it NOW!" When he is in pursuit of something he wants, this child can be so single-minded that he literally shoves his way across a room or a playground, heedless of the needs or rights of others. If he is frustrated in pursuit of his goal, he is likely to explode in tears, shrieks, and tantrums. Although these outbursts are usually short-lived, they can be so dramatic that peers come to see him as "weird" and adults may consider him emotionally disturbed.

The impatience of the ADHD child and his inability to delay gratification make it hard for him to work for long-term rewards. In the laboratory setting, as in daily life, he tends to prefer short-term payoffs, even if they are much smaller than a long-term payoff might be. Whether or not this relative insensitivity to long-term rewards should be considered a core symptom of ADHD, as some researchers argue, the practical implications are clear: in the "real world," many of the most important rewards come only after extended periods of unrewarded effort. In the long run, then, the ADHD child is at a significant disadvantage.

*Hyperactivity*

Often, but not always, inattentive children are also excessively active in situations in which they are expected to sit quietly and refrain from wiggling, fidgeting, and making noise. Many ADHD youngsters are indeed hyperactive. Variously described as "perpetually on the go," "in constant motion," and "bouncing off the walls," they exhaust their adult caretakers.

Changes in terminology have certainly contributed to confusion concerning this component of ADHD. Until 1980, the term "hyperactivity" was used to describe the syndrome. Then, in 1980, the American Psychiatric Association changed the label to "Attention Deficit Disorder." It was explicitly recognized that some inattentive, impulsive children are not excessively active, and the diagnostic category of "Attention Deficit Disorder *without* Hyperactivity" was established to include these youngsters.

In 1987, just as these new categories and terms gained widespread acceptance, there was yet another change. The diagnostic system was again revised, and once again, a new label ("Attention Deficit Hyperactivity Disorder") was coined.[#]

Unfortunately, a by-product of all of these changes has been the creation of more confusion. This confusion, in turn, has fueled a common misconception about ADHD.

**Myth All Children with ADHD Are Excessively Active.**

**Fact Children Need Not Be Hyperactive to Merit a Diagnosis of ADHD.**

Not all children who qualify for a diagnosis of ADHD are excessively active. There is a sizable subgroup of youngsters with serious attentional problems who are not at all hyperactive.[2] Some, in fact, actually appear underactive. Since their symptoms are less obvious and less troublesome to adults, these children have often been overlooked in the past. We now know that their problems—social, academic, and emotional—are as serious as those of the more classically hyperactive child.

Even among children who are quite hyperactive and disruptive, their activity level, like attentional problems, can vary considerably from one situation to another. In new or novel situations or in settings which do not demand that the child sit still and be quiet, the ADHD child may have few problems. In other settings, however, he can present a very different picture. Thus, a youngster who is quite active but generally pleasant and agreeable might be considered no problem at home or on the playground, but he may be quite a problem indeed in the classroom, where he is expected to sit quietly in his seat for long periods of time.

**ASSOCIATED PROBLEMS**

In addition to exhibiting core symptoms of ADHD, many—if not most—children with ADHD have problems in a variety of other areas. These problems include academic difficulties and learning disabilities, as well as developmental delays in speech, language, and motor skills. Coexisting psychiatric conditions such as anxiety disorders and depression are also common. In the past, many of these coexisting problems were overlooked, with the result that treatment efforts were only partially successful, at best. We now know that a diagnosis of ADHD should always alert us to the possibility of other problems, which may be more subtle but no less troublesome.

*Academic Problems and Learning Disabilities*

Children with ADHD are well known for their great difficulty with academic performance. Despite normal or even superior intelligence, the ADHD child is often a chronic underachiever. School failure is common: by adolescence, as many as one third of ADHD children have failed at least one grade in school and almost 80 percent are one or more years behind in at least one basic academic subject. Many of these youngsters are eventually placed in special education programs.

Among experts, there is general agreement concerning the overlap between ADHD and learning problems. However, researchers have disagreed on how many ADHD children have a pronounced discrepancy between their level of intelligence and the level of their academic achievement—and can therefore be considered *learning-disabled* as opposed to *learning-disordered* (see Chapter 2 for details). This disagreement is due in large part to differences in the way various researchers have defined a learning disability. Currently, researchers agree that one quarter to one third of ADHD children have at least one type of learning disability.[3]

*Speech and Language Disorders*

Children with ADHD are more likely than children in the general population to have speech and language delays and disorders. The exact figures are not known, but some researchers have found language disorders in as many as half or more of clinic-referred ADHD children.[4] Problems with expressive language are particularly likely; that is, ADHD children may have limited vocabularies, word-finding difficulties, vague and tangential speech, and poor grammar.

Language disorders, like other developmental disorders, range from mild to quite severe in degree. Although more severe forms are usually apparent by the time the child is three, in less severe forms the problems may be subtle and remain undetected for years.

What is the link between ADHD and speech/language disorders? It is apparent that as language skills develop, children are better able to express their needs through talk instead of action (for example, "Give that back" instead of a smack or a shove). Language development is also linked with the development of self-control as children come to use inner language, or "self-talk," to help them remember and abide by rules. The language-delayed child, then, may have more difficulty than others in learning to control his behavior.

It is vital that parents of a language-disordered child understand the connection between language development and behavioral self-control. Otherwise, they may place demands on the child that he cannot meet, leading to a vicious cycle of mutual frustration and anger and to escalating behavior problems.

On the other hand, parents of a language-disordered child should not assume that the child's behavioral and emotional problems stem solely from his language difficulties. If this were always the case, behavior problems would inevitably improve or disappear with improvement in language skills. This is *not* always the case, however, since research shows that almost 60 percent of youngsters with early speech/language problems continue to have emotional and/or behavioral problems as older children.[5]

The practical implications of this are clear: when a child has problems in both the language and behavior domains, a thorough evaluation of each is in order. It is only after this has been accomplished that the most appropriate treatment plan can be developed and implemented.

*Psychiatric Disorders*

Quite recently, a great deal of research has centered on the high incidence of other psychiatric disorders in children with ADHD. Among clinic-referred ADHD children, as many as half to two thirds have at least one additional psychiatric disorder. In fact, it is not uncommon for them to receive two, three, or even more diagnoses.[6]

**Oppositional Defiant Disorder and Conduct Disorder.** Among ADHD children, additional diagnoses frequently include Oppositional Defiant Disorder and Conduct Disorder. Oppositional Defiant Disorder is characterized by stubbornness, tantrums, disobedience, and defiance of authority. The oppositional child is argumentative, loses his temper easily, and blames others for his mistakes. His demeanor is such that he appears angry and resentful, often violating rules just for spite.

While the behavior of the oppositional child can drive parents to the wall, it is still less serious than that of the conduct-disordered youngster. Conduct-disordered children seem to care little about the basic rights of other people. They are often aggressive, cruel, and physically violent. During the teen years, problems with truancy, drugs, alcohol, and sexual misconduct are common. Some conduct-disordered youngsters settle down as they enter the adult years. Others, however, continue in their antisocial activities and may even graduate to criminal careers.

The well-known association between Conduct Disorder and ADHD has caused some parents to panic when their child is diagnosed with ADHD. Upon learning the diagnosis, they assume that the child is doomed to the life of a criminal or, at best, a social outcast. These parents are victims of yet another myth about ADHD.

**Myth Most ADHD Children Become Delinquents.**

**Fact ADHD and Conduct Disorder Are Separate Disorders with Different Causes and Outcomes.**

When we look at ADHD youngsters who develop serious antisocial behavior during adolescence, we find that the risk appears greatest for those who come from very dysfunctional families. Problems found in such families in- elude alcoholism and drug abuse, violence, and other kinds of antisocial behavior. Among children from intact families in which there is no history of violent or antisocial behavior, the outlook for successful adult adjustment is much better.

**Mood and Anxiety Disorders.** Since the ADHD child's life is fraught with so many difficulties and so much conflict, it is not surprising to find that problems with poor self-esteem are fairly common. What is surprising, however, is the extent to which many ADHD children actually suffer from major depression. Current research suggests that one quarter to one third of ADHD youngsters experience at least one episode of major depression during their childhood years.[7]

Children with mood disorders typically complain of sleep problems (interrupted sleep, insomnia), low energy, difficulty concentrating, feelings of chronic boredom, loss of interest in activities, and feelings of low self-esteem or of worthlessness. Changes in appetite are common, as are physical complaints, especially headaches and stomachaches. While some depressed children appear sad, withdrawn, and down-in-the-dumps, others may be grouchy, irritable, and explosive. Since there is considerable overlap between the symptoms of depression and those associated with ADHD, there is a very real possibility that the mood disorder will be overlooked and therefore go untreated.

Anxiety disorders are also more common among ADHD children than was previously suspected. Again, estimates range as high as 25 percent. Children with anxiety disorders suffer from self-consciousness and need excessive reassurance. They may fear being alone and therefore avoid separation from their parents, even when they must attend school or participate in other routine activities. It is not uncommon to find that these children have been preoccupied for years with fears and worries which they have not mentioned to their parents, in spite of a parent-child relationship which is close and loving.

Since these coexisting conditions occur so frequently among ADHD children and adults, a diagnosis of ADHD should always alert us to the possibility of their presence. If a coexisting condition goes undetected and untreated, the likelihood of a successful outcome is small indeed.

**WHAT CAUSES ADHD?**

When a child is diagnosed with ADHD, parents naturally wonder "What went wrong?" Seeking a cause for the child's difficult, unruly behavior, some parents may suspect food allergies or environmental toxins. Others blame traumatic events in the child's life, such as a move or a death in the family.

*Child-Rearing Practices*

Most commonly, parents assume that they themselves are at fault: they worry that something they have done—or something they have failed to do—has caused the problem. Unfortunately, friends, neighbors, and family members are all too often ready to agree.

**Myth The ADHD Child's Problems Reflect Poor Parenting and/or a Dysfunctional Family.**

**Fact Parents Are Not to Blame for the Primary Problems of ADHD.**

If we could peek through a keyhole to observe the patterns of interaction between ADHD children and their parents, what would we see? Dr. Russell Barkley, an eminent authority on ADHD, used one-way mirrors instead of a keyhole to observe these interactions and found that parents do tend to be controlling and negative toward their ADHD children.[8] But Dr. Barkley also found that, compared with the way in which other youngsters interacted with their parents, ADHD children were considerably more negative and disobedient. This led him to speculate that the interaction between ADHD children and their parents might be a two-way street; that is, the parents' behavior might be at least partially shaped by the children's behavior. In subsequent studies, he went on to demonstrate that when medication produced positive changes in child behavior, there was an immediate corresponding change in parent behavior. These findings certainly suggest that many parents of ADHD children actually learn to be overly controlling as a means of managing their children's difficult behavior.

Does this mean that child-rearing practices have no impact at all on the behavior of children with ADHD? Certainly not! We know that child-rearing tactics which are excessively harsh and punitive—or, conversely, too lax—only make a bad situation worse. The prognosis for the ADHD child is also less favorable when the family is disrupted by drug or alcohol problems, violence, or criminal behavior. On the other hand, parents who set clear, consistent limits and who dispense appropriate consequences for behavior provide a firm foundation for good development.

*Prenatal Problems and Birth Injuries*

Following the encephalitis epidemic of 1918, when many people who recovered from the disease were found to be unusually impulsive, active, and distractible, the notion that brain damage caused ADHD gained support. Researchers, looking for probable causes of brain damage, then turned their attention to damage which occurred during the birth process. We now believe, however, that birth injuries associated with difficult labor and fetal distress play a negligible role in ADHD.

On the other hand, the evidence does suggest that damage prior to birth may render children vulnerable to a variety of disorders, including ADHD. We know, for example, that mothers of ADHD children are more likely to have been in poor health during pregnancy. They also more frequently report suffering from preeclampsia, a serious condition characterized by high blood pressure, fluid retention, and protein in the urine. (If not treated, preeclampsia can progress to coma or convulsions and can result in maternal or fetal death.) We know, too, that mothers who abuse alcohol or drugs during pregnancy give birth to babies who suffer from a variety of problems, including ADHD and learning disabilities. Again, however, it is likely that prenatal damage accounts for only a small percentage of ADHD children.

*Environmental Toxins and Allergies*

Among the hazardous substances in our environment, lead has been the most studied in terms of its effects on human beings. In fact, lead poisoning has repeatedly been suggested as a possible cause of ADHD, but researchers have been stymied by problems in measuring lead levels in the body and by the question "How much is too much?" Although we still cannot draw firm conclusions, it is likely that lead is not the source of ADHD for most children.

Lead, of course, is not the only potentially toxic substance in our environment. As Americans have become more aware of environmental hazards, there has been increasing wariness about the possible dangers of artificial flavors, dyes, preservatives, and other food additives. In fact, one of the most widespread myths about ADHD concerns the role of diet and allergies in ADHD and learning disabilities.

**Myth Food Allergies and Poor Diet Are the Primary Causes of ADHD.**

**Fact The Relationship Between Diet and ADHD Has Not Been Consistently Demonstrated.**

Dr. Benjamin Feingold was among the first to draw widespread attention to the idea that allergic reactions to certain foods and food additives cause ADHD. Others who have followed in Dr. Feingold's footsteps include Dr. Lendon Smith and, more recently, Dr. Doris Rapp. Dr. Smith, whose theories became well known through his books *Improving Your Child's Behavior Chemistry*,[9] and *Feed Your Kids Right*,[10] argued that junk food and refined sugar cause ADHD and other behavior problems in children. Dr. Rapp, who has described her approach in television appearances and in books like *Is This Your Child?*[11] believes that unrecognized allergies to food and common environmental substances are the principal cause of these problems.

The appeal of these theories is undeniable in an era when health-conscious people watch their diets closely. As we will discuss in Chapter 7, however, when these approaches are subjected to close scientific scrutiny, we find that supporting evidence is quite meager indeed concerning the majority of children with ADHD and learning disabilities.

*Heredity*

Does ADHD "run in families" like diabetes and other disorders with a genetic component? In many families, this certainly seems to be the case. In comparison with other children, ADHD children are *four times* more likely to have close family members with the same problem. Adopted children who have ADHD are more likely to resemble their biological parents than their adoptive parents in this respect. When we examine twins, we find that identical twins are much more likely to share ADHD than fraternal (nonidentical) twins or other, nontwin siblings.

Not all cases of ADHD can be explained by heredity, nor can we predict the likelihood or severity of problems from family history alone. Nevertheless, the evidence for genetic factors as a major cause of ADHD is quite strong. But what is it that the child inherits? New research on the brain and behavior, discussed in the following section, suggests some answers to this question.

### The Brain and Behavior

Although the basic structure of the brain in the ADHD child appears to be intact (that is, there are no obvious malformations or missing pieces), this does not rule out the possibility of more subtle deviations in brain function. Because the brain is an incredibly complex organ, composed of billions of cells, even subtle deviations can account for dramatic differences in behavior. Within the past few years, increasing technological sophistication has enabled scientists to study these more subtle malfunctions.

The most recent, and most promising, approaches to the study of brain function in ADHD children have employed brain-imaging techniques. These highly sophisticated techniques not only allow us to see the structure of the brain, but they actually let us observe the brain at work.

One such technique involves measuring blood flow in different areas of the brain as a means of determining which areas are most active during different kinds of activities. This technique employs minute amounts of radioactive tracer substances which circulate through the brain and are then detected with computerized tomography (CT). Working with a group of ADHD children, scientists in Denmark found reduced blood flow in the frontal areas of the brain in every child they examined.[12] This finding is particularly exciting, since scientists have long known that the frontal lobes of the brain play a critical role in regulating attention, activity, and emotional reactions.

In the United States, Dr. Alan Zametkin, a psychiatrist at the National Institute of Mental Health, studied brain activity in adults with ADHD using a brain-imaging technique known as "PET scan."[13] The term "PET" stands for "positron emission tomography," a technique which uses a radioactive tracer substance mixed with glucose. When the brain takes up the glucose and utilizes it as fuel, the most active parts of the brain use the largest amounts of glucose. Using devices to detect the radioactive tracer substance, Dr. Zametkin compared activity in the frontal regions of the brain of ADHD subjects with that of non-ADHD individuals when both groups were told to concentrate on a task. In comparison with non-ADHD individuals, ADHD subjects had much less activity in the frontal regions of the brain.

Dr. Zametkin and other scientists believe that this pattern of frontal underactivity during concentration is due to abnormalities in the neurotransmitters (chemical messengers) in the frontal areas. They speculate that stimulant medication compensates for neurotransmitter abnormalities in these regions, thereby producing improvements in concentration and behavior. This hypothesis is supported by the finding that when treated with stimulant medication, ADHD subjects show increased activity in frontal areas which were previously underaroused.

**HOW IS ADHD DIAGNOSED?**

When parents recall the development of their ADHD children, some report that the child was excessively active even prior to birth. Some also describe a child who was fussy and difficult from the start, while others recall boundless energy and intolerance of any kind of confinement. Although these early patterns may serve to alert us to the possibility of ADHD, there is no single behavior problem which predicts ADHD with absolute certainty.

In a similar vein, parents are often surprised to learn that there is no single diagnostic procedure which serves as a litmus test for ADHD. Although there are checklists, computerized tasks, and brain-wave measurement techniques which have been billed as "surefire" ways of diagnosing ADHD, none of these techniques are without problems and limitations.

Instead, the diagnosis of ADHD involves the careful collection and analysis of information from a variety of sources. The areas in which information must be gathered in evaluating a youngster in whom ADHD is suspected are summarized below:

- History. A history of long-standing problems with attention, impulsivity, and excessive activity is the single best source of diagnostic information concerning ADHD. Family history is also important, since we know that there is a hereditary component in ADHD.

- School behavior. It is essential to obtain reports from teachers concerning the child's ability to finish work, abide by rules, and respect authority in the classroom. Since it is usually the school setting in which the ADHD child's problems are most glaringly apparent, it would be unusual indeed to find an ADHD child who was not experiencing a variety of problems in school.

- Academic achievement. In light of the relationship between ADHD and learning difficulties, it is important to assess the level of academic achievement in a child in whom ADHD is suspected.

- Intelligence. Assessment for ADHD should include at least a screening of general intelligence to rule out subaverage intellectual functioning. Children who are below average in this regard are more likely to be bewildered and frustrated by the complex demands of daily life at home and in school, so we must be sure that their symptoms truly reflect ADHD rather than frustration.

- Emotional adjustment. Since depression and anxiety disorders often coexist with ADHD, exploration of a child's emotional status is necessary to rule out these conditions. Even though an ADHD child may not be clinically depressed, information about his emotional concerns can be very useful in formulating a comprehensive treatment plan.

- Peer relations. Learning to make and keep friends is an important developmental task. Although many ADHD youngsters have no problems with it, a significant number do fare poorly. Again, information about poor social relationships can be useful in developing a good treatment plan.

- Child-rearing practices. Although child-rearing practices do not cause the primary symptoms of ADHD, how parents manage their ADHD child can make the problems much better—or much worse. It is important, too, for parents to understand how aspects of their own temperaments and personalities affect parent-child interaction and child behavior.

- Medical history and evaluation. Although it is rare that other medical problems result in symptoms which mimic ADHD, the physician must be certain to rule out a physical disorder as the source of the problem. As a rule, however, there is no need for a full neurological evaluation or an electroencephalogram (EEG) unless the physician suspects epilepsy.

*Rating Scales and Assessment Devices*

As you can see, much of the information needed to make a diagnosis of ADHD is obtained from the initial interview with the parents. In addition, information must be obtained from teachers and other significant adults in the child's life. Rating scales are an excellent way to obtain a great deal of this information in an efficient manner. They also allow us to compare a child's behavior with that of other children. By examining a child's scores on standardized rating scales, the professional can say, for example, "In terms of attention, your child has a lower rating than those achieved by 95 percent of children his age." Although there are a number of good rating scales currently available, space permits review of only a few of them here. The best-known and most widely used rating scale for assessing inattentive, hyperactive behavior in the school setting is the Conners Teacher Rating Scale. This scale was developed by Dr. Keith Conners, a psychologist now on the faculty at Duke University. Teachers are asked to rate a child on several aspects of behavior, such as "Restless or overactive" and "Disturbs other children." There is a twenty-eight-item form of this scale, as well as an abbreviated ten-item form.

A rating scale which provides a more fine-grained analysis of behavior in the school setting is the ADD-H Comprehensive Teacher Rating Scale (ACTeRS). This scale, which was standardized by administering it to teachers of more than thirty-five hundred children in kindergarten through eighth grade, allows for separate evaluation of four areas of child behavior. It is helpful not only in making an initial diagnosis of ADHD but also in monitoring response to treatment, especially with medication.

Other rating scales which can provide a great deal of helpful information include the School Situations Questionnaire and the Achenbach Child Behavior Checklist. Both of these rating scales also allow us to pinpoint specific areas in which the child encounters the greatest difficulty.

Rating scales have also been developed to assess the child's behavior in the home setting. The most widely used of these scales are the Conners Parent Rating Scale, the parent form of the Achenbach Child Behavior Checklist, and the Home Situations Questionnaire.

**Performance Tests.** When parents inquire about an evaluation of a child with attentional problems, many begin by stating, "I would like to have him tested for ADHD." They are usually somewhat surprised and disappointed to discover that there is no one test which can determine the presence or absence of ADHD.

There are, however, some performance tests which can be used to assess a youngster's ability to sustain and focus attention, as well as his ability to refrain from responding in an impulsive fashion. One such test is the Matching Familiar

Figures Test (MFFT), developed by Dr. Jerome Kagan at Harvard University.[14] In this test, the child is shown a "target" picture along with a set of similar pictures from which he must find the exact match for the target picture. In comparison with other children, ADHD children typically respond more quickly (impulsively) and make more errors before finding a match.

Another test which can shed some light on attention and impulse control is the Continuous Performance Test (CPT). The child's task here is to watch a screen on which letters or numbers are presented continuously, each appearing briefly, and to respond only to specific "target" items. One version of the CPT which has become widely available in the past few years is the Gordon Diagnostic System, which features tasks suitable for adults as well as children.[15] Another promising version of the CPT is the Test of Variables of Attention (TOVA).[16] Like the Gordon, the TOVA is a visual continuous performance task. It was designed to be used with a personal computer in the mental health professional's office, and has been standardized for children ages 6 to 18, as well as for young adults.

Although these tests can provide useful information, they are not infallible, despite their "scientific" appearance. The results must be interpreted in the context of all available information, and a diagnosis of ADHD should not be made or ruled out solely on the basis of performance on these tests.

\* The fourth edition of the *Diagnostic and Statistical Manual of Mental Disorders* (DSM-IV) is scheduled for publication in 1994. The term "Attention Deficit Hyperactivity Disorder" (ADHD) will continue to be used to describe children who are inattentive, impulsive, and hyperactive. The term "Attention Deficit Disorder" (ADD) will be used to describe children with attentional problems who are *not* hyperactive or impulsive.

# It isn't over yet! As we noted, a new edition of the *Diagnostic and Statistical Manual of Mental Disorders* is scheduled for publication in 1994. Changes in terminology will be minimal this time.

# Chapter 2

### What Are Learning Disabilities?

Despite massive expenditures on public education, illiteracy is still a serious problem in our society. A recent survey reported that 23 million people in the work force cannot read or write well enough to compete in the job market. Another study found that fewer than half of all high school graduates could compute the change that would be received from $3.00 for two items ordered from a lunch menu.[1]

In the past, when children had difficulty learning in school, they simply dropped out and entered the labor force or went to work on the family farm. Those who remained in school were often lumped together with children who were blind, deaf, mentally retarded, or emotionally disturbed. They were then segregated in separate classrooms and even separate schools. In some cases, placement in special education amounted to little more than "warehousing" the child.

This situation has changed dramatically in the past few decades as we have come to see formal education as crucial for success in life. Today, parents are not willing to accept the explanation that their children are "lazy," nor will they allow them to be isolated from their peers and placed in special classes. In increasing numbers, parents are demanding individualized programs and special services, provided in a mainstream setting.

As a result, the learning disability category has become the fastest-growing category within special education. In the past decade, the number of children identified by the schools as learning-disabled has risen from 1 percent of the school-age population to 5 percent. Funds spent on special education services for learning-disabled children have increased from 5 percent of funds distributed by the Office of Special Education Programs in 1978 to almost 50 percent in 1990.[2]

There has also been a dramatic increase in funding for research in learning disabilities. In 1980, the National Institute of Child Health and Human Development spent $2.9 million on projects related to reading disorders. In 1990, the amount spent was $7.7 million. A particularly exciting development has been the establishment of three learning disabilities research centers. Located at Yale University, Johns Hopkins University, and the University of Colorado, these centers bring together scientists from many disciplines to collaborate on research on all aspects of learning disabilities. These efforts have already begun to bear fruit in the form of increased knowledge about the causes of learning disorders and the most effective methods for treating them.

**WHO IS THE LEARNING-DISABLED CHILD?**

How do you recognize a child who has learning disabilities? As Sally Smith[3] has so aptly pointed out, there are "no easy answers," but often we find that the learning-disabled youngster is one who:

- Can recite the batting average of every player in the American League since 1952 but cannot remember the names of his classmates.

- Reads "saw" for "was," "god" for "dog," and "dog" for "doughnut," so that what he thinks he has read bears no relationship to what is actually on the page in front of him.

- Is very verbal and reads voraciously but subtracts 7 from 12 and comes up with 15.

- Earns scores in the superior range on intelligence tests but balks at doing even minimum amounts of written work.

Confronted with a child like this, parents vacillate between scratching their heads and tearing out their hair. How, they wonder, can he sound so smart and act so dumb? How can he be so bright yet perform so abysmally in the classroom?

What's wrong with these children? Are they, as one controversial book[4] suggests, able-minded underachievers who have the ability but not the "will" to do the work? Do they suffer from psychological problems which result in "work inhibition"? Are they just lazy?

**LEARNING DISABILITIES DEFINED**

It is a safe bet that there is at least as much confusion surrounding the term "learning disability" as there is about the term "hyperactivity." Certainly, it is an area in which myths and misunderstandings abound.

Part of the confusion stems from the way in which learning disabilities are defined. The term "learning-disabled" refers only to *children who fail to learn despite an apparently normal capacity for learning.* This means that not all children who perform poorly in school can be considered learning-disabled. For example, a child whose academic performance is deficient because he is blind, deaf, or paralyzed is not considered learning-disabled, nor do we use the term to refer to a child whose learning difficulties stem from a generally low level of intelligence (mental retardation) or severe environmental deprivation.

In 1975, Public Law 94-142, the Education for All Handicapped Children Act, was passed. This law provided the following definition of a learning disability: "Specific learning disability means a disorder in one or more of the basic ... processes involved in understanding or in using language, spoken or written. [This may take the form of] imperfect ability to listen, think, speak, read, write, spell or do mathematical calculations."

Federal guidelines state that in order for a child to be considered learning-disabled, there must be a significant discrepancy between the child's potential for learning (as assessed by intelligence tests) and his actual academic achievement in one or more of seven areas. These include:

· Oral expression (speaking)

- Listening comprehension (understanding)

- Written expression

- Basic reading

- Reading comprehension

- Mathematics calculation

- Mathematics reasoning (problem solving)

On the face of it, this approach to defining learning disabilities appears straightforward. Unfortunately, since the magnitude of the discrepancy was not specified in the federal guidelines, all sorts of misunderstandings and confusion have followed. Should we consider a 10-point difference between intelligence test scores and achievement test scores a "discrepancy"? A 20-point difference? If the child is a year behind his peers in reading, is this a "significant" delay? Or should we insist that he be two or more years behind in order for him to be considered learning- disabled?

Quibbling over the fine points of a definition may seem like nit-picking, but the way in which we define learning disabilities has very important implications for determining who is eligible to receive remedial and support services. Too restrictive a definition will result in denying these services to children who truly need them. On the other hand, if we define the condition too loosely, we will include many normal learners who do not need special education services. Since these services are costly, this will put an impossible fiscal strain on school systems at a time when schools throughout the country are facing budget cutbacks.

Researchers, too, need a clear definition of learning disabilities. Lack of agreement concerning a definition has made it difficult to interpret research results and to compare findings from one study to the next. This has caused no end of confusion when researchers have tried to estimate prevalence rates (since rates vary widely depending on the definition used), identify associated problems, and determine what kinds of treatment programs are most effective.

Currently, the most widely accepted approach to defining a learning disability calls for a discrepancy of at least 20 points between intelligence test scores and achievement test scores. Using this definition, it is estimated that learning disabilities occur in about 10 percent of the U.S. population. Learning disabilities affect boys and girls in approximately equal numbers, although more boys than girls are referred for help. The reason for this remains unclear: perhaps boys are more severely affected or, as some have suggested, are more disruptive and troublesome to parents and teachers.

**SPECIFIC LEARNING DISABILITIES**

Researchers have used all kinds of classification schemes to categorize and study different types of learning disabilities. Some, for example, have categorized learning disabilities on the basis of specific processes which they think are involved in learning. These include visual and auditory perception, sequencing, visual-motor integration, and memory processes.

For the purpose of our discussion, we have simply divided learning disabilities into two broad groups: 1) those which involve auditory-verbal processes, resulting in reading disorders and other language-based learning problems; and 2) those which involve visual and motor (nonverbal) processes, resulting in poor handwriting, difficulties in mathematics, and deficits in certain social skills. Table 2 provides an overview of the areas of learning and achievement which are affected by each set of skills.

*Reading Disorders and Other Language-Based Learning Disabilities*

Reading disorders, often referred to collectively as "dyslexia," are by far the most common of the learning disabilities, accounting for the vast majority of all referrals for diagnosis and remediation. They are generally the most troublesome as well, with consequences which are more pervasive and far-reaching than those of other kinds of learning disorders. Sloppy handwriting, weak math skills, and poor coordination may have only mild nuisance value in daily life, especially in the adult years. Many otherwise competent and successful people cannot balance a checkbook or catch a baseball, but these deficits have little impact on their overall ability to function in society.

Poor reading ability, on the other hand, can cause significant life problems not only during the school years but well past the time an individual leaves formal schooling behind. Reading skills are important in everyday life. And although reading disorders certainly do not preclude success in adult years, they continue to present practical problems in many aspects of personal and professional life.

Finally, reading disorders are the most misunderstood of the learning disabilities. It is ironic—and unfortunate—that the public continues to be bombarded with misinformation about reading disorders, since we actually know a great deal about the specific skill deficits associated with them.

**Skill Deficits in Reading Disorders.** A host of explanations have been advanced for reading disorders, including faulty eye movements, problems with visual perception or coordination between visual and motor functions, failure of the eyes to work together, and so on. These theories have given rise to one of the most common misconceptions about dyslexia.

Myth Dyslexia Is Caused by Problems with Visual-Spatial Functions.

Fact Dyslexia Is Due to Impaired Language- Processing Skills.

It is not difficult to understand why this myth is so widespread. The connection between the eyes and reading is an obvious one (try reading with your eyes closed!), and in fact, there are differences between good and poor readers in the patterns of eye movement during reading. Many poor readers also have difficulty with reversals, confusing the letters "b" and "d," for example, and reading "was" as "saw."

*Table 2*

| | | | **Auditory-Verbal** | | |
|---|---|---|---|---|---|
| Conceptual | | | Verbal Conceptual | | |
| Rote/ Automatic | Auditory Motor | Auditory Perceptual | Rote Auditory Sequential Memory | Rote and Association Memory and Retrieval | |

| | | **Visual-Motor** | | |
|---|---|---|---|---|
| Conceptual | | Visual/Nonverbal Conceptual | | |
| Rote/ Automatic | Letter Perception | Spatial Organization and Nonverbal Integration | Rote Visual/Sequential Memory and Retrieval | Motor Sequencing/Fine Motor Control |

—Sally Ingalls, Ph.D.
Neurology, Learning and Behavior Center © 1991

Research evidence, however, clearly indicates that reading-disabled individuals actually have impaired language-processing skills, especially in what are called "phonological processes." As Dr. Bruce Pennington, a prominent neuropsychologist at the University of Denver, explains:

> Over and over again when we read, we must translate printed letter strings into word pronunciations. To do this, we must understand that the alphabet is a code for phonemes, the individual speech sounds in the language, and we must be able to use that code quickly and automatically so that we can concentrate on the meaning of what we read. The difficulty that dyslexics have with "phonics," the ability to sound out words, makes reading much slower and less automatic and detracts considerably from comprehension.[5]

In addition to difficulty understanding written material, many children with reading disorders have problems understanding what they hear. Because they have problems distinguishing between similar sounds (for example, "mine" versus "mind"), their listening comprehension may be impaired, especially in a noisy environment in which other sounds compete with the main speaker.

*Levels of Processing Related to Learning Disability/Disability Characteristics*

Auditory/Verbal

**Conceptual** · Language semantics—word meaning, definition vocabulary

|  |  |
|---|---|
|  | · Listening comprehension—understanding and memory of overall ideas |
|  | · Reading comprehension—understanding and memory of overall ideas |
|  | · Specificity and variety of verbal concepts for oral or written expression |
|  | · Verbal reasoning and logic |
| **Automatic** | · Early speech—naming objects |
|  | · Auditory processing—clear enunciation of speech, pronouncing sounds/syllables in correct order |
|  | · Name colors |
|  | · Recall birthdate, phone number, address, etc. |
|  | · Say alphabet and other lists (days, months) in order |
|  | · Easily select and sequence words with proper grammatical structure for oral or written expression |
|  | · Auditory "dyslexia"—discriminate sounds, especially vowels; auditory blend sounds to words, distinguish words that sound alike, e.g., mine/mind |
|  | · Labeling and retrieval reading disorder—perceives auditory and visual okay but continually mislabels letters sounds, common syllables, sight words (b/d, her/here) |
|  | · Poor phonic spelling |
|  | · Poor listening/reading comprehension due to poor short-term memory, especially for rote facts |
|  | · Labeling and retrieval math disorder—trouble counting sequentially, mislabels numbers (16/60), poor memory for number facts and sequences of steps for computation (e.g., long division) |
|  | · Recall names, dates, and historical facts |
|  | · Learn and retain new science terminology |

## Visual/Motor

| | |
|---|---|
| **Conceptual** | · Social insight and reasoning—ability to understand strategies of games, jokes, motives of others, social conventions, tact |
| | · Math concepts—use of zero in operations; place value, money equivalences, missing elements, etc. |
| | · Inferential reading comprehension; drawing conclusions |
| | · Understanding relationship of historical events across time; understanding science concepts |
| | · Structuring ideas hierarchically; outlining skills |
| | · Generalization abilities |
| | · Integrating material into a well-organized report |
| **Automatic** | · Assembling puzzles and building with construction toys |
| | · Social perception and awareness of environment |

- Time sense—doesn't ask, "Is this the last recess?"

- Remembers and executes correct sequence for tying shoes

- Easily negotiates stairs, climbs on play equipment, learns athletic skills, and rides bike

- Can execute daily living skills such as pouring without spilling, spreading a sandwich, dressing self correctly

- Using the correct sequence of strokes to form manuscript or cursive letters

- Eye-hand coordination for drawing, assembling art project, and handwriting

- Directional stability for top/bottom and left/right tracking

- Copy from board accurately

- Visual "dyslexia"—confused when viewing visual symbols, poor visual discrimination, reversals/inversions/ transpositions due to poor directionality, may not recognize the shape or form of a word that has been seen many times before, i.e., "word-blind"

- Spelling—poor visual memory for the nonphonetic elements of words

—Sally Ingalls, Ph.D., 1990 Used with permission

Problems with verbal short-term memory are also common among dyslexic individuals because such memory requires use of phonological skills. Thus, poor readers may have problems recalling letters, digits, words, or phrases in exact sequence. When problems with verbal short-term memory occur together with poor listening comprehension, it is obvious that the individual will have particular difficulty following verbal directions, especially if he is in a noisy setting.

Table 3: Myths and Facts About Learning Disabilities

| Myth | Fact |
| --- | --- |
| Dyslexia is caused by problems with visual-spatial functions. | Dyslexia is due to impaired language-processing skills. |
| Learning disabilities are caused by allergies. | There is no evidence that treatment of allergies helps learning problems. |

**Associated Problems.** In addition to these difficulties, children with reading disorders have problems in a variety of other areas. They include the following:

*Other Academic Problems.* Deficits in auditory-verbal abilities have a marked impact on other academic skills, such as spelling, writing, and even arithmetic. In fact, among poor readers, spelling is generally even more impaired than reading ability.[6] As Dr. Pennington points out, we do not simply memorize the spelling of words. If we did, each new word we encountered would be completely novel and we could not use information from words already known. Instead, we rely on our knowledge of phonics to learn and remember the spelling of new words.[*]

Poor auditory-verbal abilities can also have an adverse effect on the production of written material, since the same coding processes are used in both reading and writing. However, writing also requires additional skills. In fact, since writing involves both automatic and conceptual verbal skills as well as motor skills, it is the most complex academic process we must master. Not only must we remember the phonological code; we must also think of the words to express what we want to say, organize them according to the rules of grammar and syntax, and then go through the mechanical process of putting them on paper —paying attention, of course, to the size, shape, and spacing of the letters, punctuation, and so on. The wonder is not that so many children have difficulty with written expression but that any of us ever learn to write at all!

Many dyslexic children also have difficulty with mathematics. They may, for example, have difficulty memorizing basic math facts and remembering sequences of steps for computation (for example, long division). They may mislabel numbers, confusing 16 with 60, and they often have difficulty understanding word problems.

*Speech and Language Problems.* Among children with reading disorders, it is common to find a history of early developmental speech and language disorders. In addition to delayed speech, problems include difficulty naming objects and colors and remembering one's address, telephone number, and the like. Problems with word retrieval (finding the right word to express one's meaning) are also common.

There is also a well-documented association between reading disorders and developmental articulation disorders. In an articulation disorder, mispronunciations occur because individual sounds are substituted, omitted, or distorted. While some cases of articulation disorders are caused by faulty hearing or structural defects in the mouth or tongue, difficulties with phonology appear to be the source of the problem for many individuals.

On the other hand, stuttering and other disorders of speech fluency are not associated with reading disorders. In these disorders, it is the rhythm of speech that is disturbed, not the pronunciation of speech sounds.

*Attention Deficit Hyperactivity Disorder.* As we discussed in Chapter 1, there is considerable overlap between learning and attention problems. We noted that when we examine a group of ADHD children, we find that approximately 19 to 26 percent also have learning disabilities. Conversely, when we begin with a group of children who have been diagnosed as dyslexic, we find that about one third also have ADHD.

What are we to make of this relationship? Researchers who have studied the question have come up with at least three theories about the link between ADHD and learning disabilities: 1) ADHD children have difficulty with academic achievement because they are inattentive and impulsive; 2) learning-disabled children "turn off and tune out" in the classroom because the work is so difficult for them; and 3) ADHD and dyslexia share a common genetic cause, so a child who inherits one disorder will also inherit the other.

After years of heated debate, it appears that all three theories have merit. In some cases, ADHD and dyslexia may occur together because of a shared genetic cause.[7] In other cases, even when there is no common genetic cause, there is a reciprocal relationship between ADHD and learning difficulties; that is, inattentive behavior leads to learning problems, and learning problems make it likely that the child will often be inattentive and off-task.[8]

*Allergic Disorders.* Many investigators have reported a high incidence of allergies in dyslexic children. This observation has given rise to one of the most common myths concerning learning disabilities.

**Myth Learning Disabilities Are Caused by Allergies.**

**Fact There Is No Evidence That Treatment of Allergies Helps Learning Problems.**

As we have explained elsewhere, simply knowing that two things are related does not explain the direction of the relationship; that is, whether A causes B, B causes A, or both A and B are due to a third cause. In the case of the relationship between allergies and learning disorders, many people have interpreted this relationship to mean that allergies *cause* learning disabilities, and have devised treatment programs designed to remediate learning problems by treating suspected allergies (see Chapter 7).

An alternative—and equally plausible—explanation of the relationship between allergies and learning disabilities is that both are caused by a third factor. In fact, recent evidence concerning genetics suggests that this is indeed the case, at least in certain types of learning disorders. At the University of Colorado, Dr. John DeFries and his colleagues have identified a subtype of hereditary dyslexia which is linked to chromosome 6. Since this chromosome contains many genes that affect the immune system, Dr. DeFries believes that there may be a gene in this region which affects both reading and immune functions.[9] If this is the case, treating one set of symptoms (allergies) would not be expected to have any effect on the second set of symptoms (reading problems).

*Emotional Disorders.* A link between learning disabilities and emotional problems has been identified by several investigators. Some, for example, have found depressive symptoms in a third or more of the learning-disabled children they studied,[10] a figure which is obviously much higher than in the general population. The most current research also suggests that different subtypes of learning disorders are associated with different kinds of emotional/psychological problems. Specifically, language-based learning disabilities appear to be related to the so-called "externalizing disorders" of ADHD and Conduct Disorder, while nonverbal learning disabilities seem to have a stronger relationship with depression and anxiety disorders, the "internalizing disorders."

From a commonsense perspective, the connection between learning disabilities and psychological problems seems obvious. After years of struggling —and failing—to perform in school, it would be quite surprising if the learning-disabled youngster were not somewhat depressed and demoralized. It seems equally apparent that a child who suffers from crippling depression and/or anxiety will have little energy available for learning.

Here again, however, we must be cautious about a chicken-and-egg approach in attributing cause to one set of problems or the other. Much time and energy may be wasted if we focus on trying to determine whether a child can't read because he is distracted by fears and worries or whether he is (justifiably) anxious because he can't perform in school. Instead, we would do far better to simply recognize the existence of both emotional and learning problems and develop a treatment plan that addresses both.

*Visual-Motor Learning Disabilities*

This group of learning disabilities includes specific problems with arithmetic and handwriting which may occur *with or without* associated reading disabilities. Also included under the heading of visual-motor learning disabilities are deficits in social awareness and social judgment. Since these problems are not language-based in nature, they are also referred to as "nonverbal learning disabilities."

Nonverbal learning disabilities occur much less frequently than language-based learning disabilities. Studies show that among children referred to learning disability clinics, only about 1 to 10 percent have nonverbal learning disabilities.

Nonverbal learning disabilities are sometimes called "right-hemisphere learning disabilities." Since there are many complex connections between the right and left hemispheres (sides) of the brain, it would be an oversimplification to speak of one hemisphere of the brain as if it existed in complete isolation from the other. In general, however, we can say that the brain is organized in such a way that the left hemisphere is specialized for language, while the right hemisphere is specialized for processing nonverbal information. This includes spatial awareness, recognition and organization of visual patterns, and coordination of visual information with motor processes (visual-motor integration). The right hemisphere is also specialized for detecting differences between tones, so it has major responsibility for perceiving melody in music as well as the melodic pattern of spoken language (variations in tone and stress).

As we might expect, children who have right-hemisphere learning disabilities are often poorly coordinated in terms of both fine and gross motor skills. They may have difficulty learning to ride a bike and mastering other athletic skills. At a preschool level, they have problems with cut-and-paste activities, using crayons and markers, and learning to tie their shoes. They are also poor at assembling puzzles and building with construction toys. As they grow older, we see weaknesses in nonverbal problem solving and concept formation. Although these children may have very well developed rote verbal memory, they have a great deal of difficulty adapting to novel or complex situations.

**Specific Deficits.** As noted, these children have difficulty in the areas of handwriting and arithmetic, often without associated reading problems. They also have problems with social awareness and judgment.

*Handwriting.* Eye-hand coordination is an obviously important factor in handwriting. The child with a right- hemisphere learning disability may have difficulty remembering the shapes of letters (poor visual memory) and using the correct sequence of strokes to form letters. He may also have an awkward pencil grip. Letters are poorly spaced and of different sizes, and writing is quite slow and labored. Copying accurately from the board is also likely to be particularly difficult for this youngster.

*Arithmetic.* The specific difficulties with arithmetic found in children with right-hemisphere learning disabilities lie in understanding the fundamental concepts of mathematics. In this regard, their problems with math are different from those seen in dyslexic children, who struggle to memorize math facts and understand word problems. Consequently, the kinds of arithmetic errors made by dyslexic children and those with specific arithmetic disability are quite different. Dyslexic children may make mistakes because they reverse numbers or forget basic math facts and have to count on their fingers, but they usually grasp the basic principles and subroutines needed to solve the problem. In contrast, the child with a specific math disability has difficulty understanding what approach is required to solve a particular problem and what a reasonable answer might be.

*Social Skills Deficits.* While there are certainly children with specific math and handwriting disabilities who do not have social difficulties, the problems overlap so frequently that social skills disabilities are considered a component of nonverbal learning disabilities.

The problems in social interaction seen in individuals with right-hemisphere learning disabilities seem to reflect difficulty in perceiving nonverbal cues in communication. Their visual-spatial-organizational deficits put them at a disadvantage in recognizing faces and interpreting gestures, body posture, and facial expressions. They also have difficulty perceiving vocal cues in spoken language, such as rate, tone, and emphasis.

These deficits place the child at a real social disadvantage because nonverbal signals and cues are so important in communication. For example, in an average conversation between two people, the verbal components carry less than 35 percent of the social meaning of the situation, while more than 65 percent is conveyed through nonverbal messages. Nonverbal behavior is especially important in communicating feelings, emotions, and liking or disliking. In fact, it is estimated that of the total liking or affection we communicate to another person, only 7 percent is actually communicated through words. Voice cues like pitch and volume carry 38 percent; facial expression and eye contact, 55 percent.[11]

Nonverbal cues also function like traffic signals to regulate conversational beginnings and endings, turn-takings in conversation, and changes in subject. Just as an automobile driver who doesn't respond to traffic signals will be considered a poor driver, so too the person who can't "read" nonverbal cues will be seen as rude, boorish, and socially inept.

*Emotional Problems.* As we mentioned earlier in this chapter, children with nonverbal learning disabilities seem particularly prone to developing so-called "internalizing disorders," characterized by depression and/or anxiety. In that section, we also alluded to questions concerning the direction of this relationship; that is, do learning disabilities cause emotional problems or do emotional problems prevent the child from learning appropriately, thereby causing learning disabilities?

A third possibility, of course, is that some other factor, such as an underlying problem within the central nervous system, actually lies at the root of both kinds of problems. Dr. Byron Rourke, an authority on nonverbal learning disabilities, believes that the evidence is strongest in favor of this last notion and thinks that a disturbance in the right hemisphere can account for both sets of problems.[12]

This reminds us once again that we should not limit ourselves to a naive either-or approach when confronted with a youngster who appears to suffer from both learning and emotional problems. Instead, we should direct our resources toward accurate diagnosis and appropriate remediation of both conditions.

**WHAT CAUSES LEARNING DISABILITIES?**

Since language-based and nonverbal learning disabilities appear to have different causes, especially in regard to the site of the problem within the brain, we will consider each category separately.

*Language-Based Learning Disabilities*

**Genetic Factors.** Almost from the time dyslexia was first described, early in this century, heredity has been known to play an important role. Heredity probably accounts for the majority of language-based learning disabilities, and when we look at family members of individuals with dyslexia, we usually find that 35 to 40 percent of their closest relatives have similar difficulties. In some families, dyslexia is linked to genetic markers on chromosome 15,[13] while in others, chromosome 6 appears to be involved.[14]

**Environmental Factors.** We know less about environmental causes of dyslexia than we do about genetic factors. As is the case with ADHD, there is a link between learning disorders and maternal alcohol abuse during pregnancy. Mothers who abuse "crack" cocaine give birth to babies who suffer from a variety of problems, including ADHD and learning disabilities. The link with maternal smoking is less clear: mothers who smoke give birth to smaller babies, but since woman who smoke during pregnancy often abuse alcohol as well, it may be that alcohol is the critical factor in the relationship.

Some researchers have also implicated environmental toxins and pollutants, but this link is also difficult to confirm. Others have reported a relationship between reading disorders and both large family size and low socioeconomic status.[15] In large families, it is more difficult for all children to receive optimal amounts of attention and stimulation; in some impoverished families, parents do not spend much time reading to their children or playing language games with them.

**Brain Mechanisms in Dyslexia.** Researchers generally agree that dyslexia involves dysfunction in the left hemisphere of the brain, the hemisphere which is specialized for language. Using brain-imaging techniques like PET scans, scientists have consistently found differences in left-hemisphere functioning in dyslexics, even with tasks that do not involve reading.

One area in particular, known as the *"planum temporale,"* has been the focus of recent promising research. In most people, this area is asymmetrical, with the area on the left side of the brain larger than that on the right side. In dyslexics, however, researchers have found that these areas are equal in size (symmetrical) or that the right side is actually larger than the left. At Harvard University Medical School, for example, Dr. Albert Galaburda and his colleagues have performed autopsies on the brains of ten dyslexic individuals and have found this pattern in every case.[16] Their findings have also been supported by the results of studies in which magnetic resonance imaging (MRI) techniques have been used to compare the brains of dyslexics and nondyslexic individuals.[17]

Neuroscientists are not certain what causes this difference. One possibility is that during early development of the brain, some cells migrate to the wrong areas. Other possibilities include overproduction of brain cells in certain areas and failure of the system to "prune" (remove) excess brain cells. According to Dr. Galaburda, factors that control production of brain cells are likely to be mainly genetic, while "pruning" depends on environmental influences as well as genetic factors. This would account for the fact that some cases of dyslexia appear to be hereditary in origin, while environmental factors may be important in others.

*Visual-Motor Learning Disabilities*

**Genetic Factors.** No family studies of these disorders have been done, so we have very little information about the role of heredity in the nonverbal learning disabilities. However, we do know that two specific genetic syndromes, Turner syndrome and Fragile X syndrome in females, are associated with specific problems in arithmetic, handwriting, and social skills.[18]

**Environmental Factors.** In Boston, the eminent neurologist Marcel Mesulam studied fourteen children with nonverbal learning disabilities and found evidence of brain damage in nine of them.[19] At the University of Windsor, Dr. Byron Rourke and his associates found nonverbal learning disabilities in children who suffered moderate to severe head injuries; children who had received radiation treatment of the head; children who had been unsuccessfully treated for hydrocephalus; and children who had significant amounts of tissue removed from the right hemisphere. Since all of these conditions involve destruction of white matter (the long, myelinated fibers in the brain) in the right hemisphere, Dr. Rourke believes that nonverbal learning disabilities are caused by early damage to white matter in the right hemisphere.

## HOW ARE LEARNING DISABILITIES DIAGNOSED?

The process by which learning disabilities are diagnosed stems directly from the specific questions the evaluator is asked to address. If, for example, the question is "Does this child read as well as expected for his age and grade?" the evaluator can use standardized tests which enable him to derive age and grade scores for the child's level of achievement. Tests like the Woodcock-Johnson Psychoeducational Battery[20] and the Peabody Individual Achievement Test[21] are reliable and efficient tools for this purpose. These tests assess specific academic skills such as word and sentence reading, reading comprehension, vocabulary, spelling, math knowledge, and math application. Because these tests are administered on an individual basis, they are often very helpful with inattentive or learning-disabled children to accurately assess their levels of achievement. Often individual testing avoids many of the problems encountered by inattentive and learning-disabled children during group testing. Individual assessment also allows the evaluator to take additional time to build motivation and make certain that the best possible performance is being obtained. Tests such as these are well standardized. *Standardization* refers to the process by which a test is administered to thousands of children across the country in an effort to provide a sample of children which recognizes the contribution of differences such as age, sex, educational experience, socioeconomic status, and even ethnic background.

But there are additional steps which go beyond simply ascertaining whether the child reads at a level commensurate with his age and grade level. For example, we might also ask "Does this child read as well as would be expected on the basis of his level of general intelligence?" This question is usually asked when an administrative decision must be made about the child's eligibility to receive special services through the public school system. To answer this question, the evaluator uses a standardized intelligence test ("IQ test") such as the Wechsler Intelligence Scale for Children[22] or the cognitive component of the Woodcock-Johnson Psychoeducational Battery. Such tests must be administered on an individual basis by someone who has been specifically trained to administer them and to score and interpret the results. They are somewhat costly to administer, therefore, and school systems are generally reluctant to offer them unless there is good reason to suspect a real discrepancy between a child's intelligence and his academic achievement.

There is still another level of assessment, which involves identifying the particular skill deficits and areas of weakness which underlie a child's learning problems. To address this issue, evaluators use a variety of psychological and neuropsychological tests, such as the Halstead-Reitan Battery for Children or the Luria Nebraska Child and Adolescent Test Battery. In addition, they observe the child as he works with academic tasks so that they can make qualitative judgments about his performance. Thus, in addition to obtaining a child's age and grade scores in reading, for example, the evaluator actually listens to the child read in order to pinpoint specific strengths and weaknesses.

This information is then combined with other information about the child's behavior, attention, motivation, motor skills, speech and language abilities, and so on, to arrive at a comprehensive understanding of the child's functioning. Ideally, such a comprehensive assessment should lead logically to specific intervention strategies to remedy the problems and improve the child's ability to achieve. These strategies will be reviewed in Chapter 5.

\* Some children with good visual memory skills can compensate for poor phonetic ability. They may struggle to spell unfamiliar words, but once a word is learned, they remember it. As you can see, some children are capable of compensating for a weakness in one skill area with a strength in another.

# SECTION II
# Effective Treatments for ADHD and Learning Disabilities

## Chapter 3

How New Treatments Are Evaluated: Science, Pseudoscience, and Quackery

The word "science" usually calls up images of a laboratory in which white-coated technicians do mysterious things with beakers of chemicals and turn dials on complicated instruments and machines. But psychologists and others who study human behavior are also scientists. Along with physicists and chemists, they believe that the *scientific method* is the best way to go about answering questions about everything—from why people behave as they do to why protons and electrons "behave" as they do.

As intimidating as it sounds, the scientific method is really nothing more than a set of rules about how evidence should be gathered and evaluated in order to answer a specific question or solve a specific problem. As the eminent philosopher and mathematician Bertrand Russell explained, "It is not *what* the man of science believes that distinguishes him, but *how* and *why* he believes it. His beliefs are tentative, not dogmatic; they are based on evidence, not authority."[1]

In this chapter, we will explain how the scientific method is used to evaluate new treatments for children with ADHD and learning disabilities. We will then compare this approach with the way in which new treatments for these problems are presented to the public.

### THE PROCESS OF SCIENTIFIC INVESTIGATION

The process by which a particular treatment is scientifically evaluated is longer and more arduous than most of us realize. It begins with a question or idea, phrased as a hypothesis. This hypothesis is usually based on an existing body of knowledge. An example might be: "Since stimulant medication helps children with ADHD, it might also help ADHD adolescents."

The second step in the process is the development of a research program, or protocol, to test the hypothesis. The treatment itself, the way in which it will be implemented, and the group of people to whom it will be applied must all be carefully defined. Thus, the researcher must specify exactly how much medication will be given to how many patients for what period of time. He must also clearly describe the way in which the people he will study, called "subjects," are to be selected. In the example above, for instance, it is not sufficient to say only that teenagers with ADHD will be studied. The investigator must also describe other characteristics of his subjects, such as age and intelligence, and he must identify the diagnostic tests and procedures used to make the diagnosis of ADHD.

*Ruling Out Alternative Explanations*

The researcher must also specify the way in which the treatment will be evaluated. Care must be taken to ensure that the results he obtains are really due to the treatment under study rather than to some other factor unrelated to the treatment.

An example from the physical sciences illustrates the importance of ruling out alternative explanations for results. In the early 1960s, Russian scientists claimed to have discovered a new form of water with strange, nonwaterlike properties.[2] This liquid, which came to be called "polywater," resulted when ordinary water was sealed in glass tubes for a few days. Polywater did not boil at 100 degrees Celsius, and when it froze, it formed a solid that was not ice. Although some skeptics contended that polywater was nothing more than normal water which had somehow become contaminated with impurities, researchers repeatedly failed to find any impurities.

By the mid-1960s, ten scientific papers had been published and the mass media took note, touting polywater as the most important chemical discovery of the century. Concern grew about the potential dangers of polywater if it were to be accidently released into general water supplies, and the military began to explore the use of polywater as an offensive weapon. It was not until the mid-1970s, after the publication of 115 research studies and 112 articles in the popular press, that scientists agreed that polywater resulted from nothing more than contaminants in the quartz tubes in which it was contained. In fact, no polymer of water had been discovered at all.

**Placebo Effects and the Power of Suggestion.** When scientists study human behavior, they must take particular care to eliminate the placebo effect as an alternative explanation of their results. Placebo, which is Latin for "I shall please," refers to the well-documented fact that people may respond to all sorts of ineffective treatments as long as they believe that the treatments have the power to help them.

The use of placebo and suggestion in the treatment of human ailments is by no means new. At the dawn of civilization, high priests used elaborate ceremonies and rituals to heighten the sufferer's expectation of relief and recovery. These methods were sometimes surprisingly effective, as evidenced by the awe in which priests and shamans were held and by their power and status in society.

Placebo effects can be more powerful than most people realize. In a classic example, a drug known to cause vomiting actually brought relief to people suffering from severe nausea and vomiting when they were told it would help them.[3] In another study, if people were given a sedative and told that it would energize them, they responded with increased energy and arousal. If, on the other hand, they were given a stimulant which they were told was a sedative, they became sleepy and reacted as if they had actually taken a sedative. Even a drug as potent as morphine has a placebo effect: among patients suffering from postoperative pain, about 75 percent obtain significant relief from morphine. However, about 35 percent obtain a comparable degree of relief from a sugar solution, which suggests that about half of the effect of morphine may be a placebo effect.[4]

Exactly how does a placebo work? No one knows the answer to this question, but we do know that the tendency to respond to a placebo does not depend on a personality trait like "suggestibility" or "dependency." Instead, an individual's response is influenced by various aspects of the specific situation. For example, if the professional who provides the treatment is enthusiastic in his endorsement of the treatment, the placebo effect is enhanced. It is also heightened if the professional is seen as trustworthy and caring, particularly if he is someone in a position of status or authority. Finally, we can expect a greater placebo effect if the treatment involves impressive high-tech equipment and complicated procedures.

The placebo effect is usually considered a nuisance by researchers because it complicates the process of evaluating new drugs and procedures. Since suggestion, even in its subtlest form, can have such powerful effects, the use of the so-called "double-blind" technique is essential in the evaluation of new treatments. When the double-blind technique is used, neither the subject nor the researcher knows whether the patient has received the real ("active") treatment or the placebo treatment. Otherwise, the expectations of either or both could seriously bias the results.

Double-blind procedures are relatively simple when the treatment under investigation consists of a pill or a capsule. Placebo pills, identical in appearance to the active drug, are made up and placed in coded containers. This code is not revealed to the researchers, who work directly with the subjects until the end of the study, after all evaluations have been completed.

When the treatment under study involves not a pill but a procedure, such as a controlled diet or a training program, it is more difficult to devise a placebo treatment and to use the double-blind technique. Often, under these conditions, researchers must exercise a great deal of ingenuity to come up with a placebo procedure which is equivalent to the active procedure. In the case of a diet study, for example, they must create a placebo diet that is as convincing as the diet actually under study so that the subjects who participate in the investigation cannot distinguish between the two.

*Evaluating the Results*

Even after all of this careful planning, the researcher is not ready to begin his investigation until he has nailed down the technical details about how he will measure and analyze the results of the treatment. This can be a complicated issue because when we study human behavior, many of the things we want to measure cannot be physically quantified. We can't weigh "hyperactivity" on a scale, nor do we have a yardstick by which to measure "aggression." Therefore, investigators must describe exactly what they will observe and how they will measure it. One measure of hyperactivity, for example, might be the number of times a child leaves his seat in a ten-minute period. Measures of attention and concentration often include scores on continuous performance tests such as the Gordon Diagnostic System and the Test of Variables of Attention, as well as such "real world" measures as the amount of time a child remains on-task while doing academic work.

Finally, the researcher must stipulate how he will analyze the measurements so that he can say with some degree of certainty that any improvements observed are really due to his treatment rather than to chance fluctuations. To do this, he uses statistical tests to compare the scores of subjects who received the active treatment with those of subjects who received the placebo treatment. If the difference between the treatment and placebo groups' scores is so great that the results could be expected to occur by chance only once or so in a hundred trials, the researcher is justified in concluding that the difference is "statistically significant" (that is, it is unlikely to be a chance occurrence, so the difference between the active treatment and the placebo treatment is probably a real difference).

In evaluating treatments designed to help children with ADHD and learning disabilities, statistical significance may not be enough: we also need to know whether the results are *clinically significant*. For example, a particular treatment might produce statistically significant improvements in scores on laboratory tests such as building block towers or recalling lists of words, but it might have no real effect on performance in the home or school setting. Such a treatment might be of interest to scientists seeking to understand the nature of ADHD or learning disabilities, but it would be of little interest or value to parents who want to obtain help for their child.

### The Final Product

After the experiment has been completed and the results analyzed, the findings must be subjected to the scrutiny of other researchers so that the entire scientific community can evaluate the work. This means that the findings must be published in journals which accept articles only after peer review; that is, after other scientists with expertise in the same field have reviewed the work and determined that it meets standards of scientific acceptability.

After all of this, you would certainly think that our conscientious researcher, worn out from his painstaking efforts, could rest on his laurels and bask in the glory of having answered an important question about human behavior. Right? Wrong! Few experiments—very few indeed—produce results which are so clear-cut and compelling that all questions about the treatment are answered once and for all. In reality, no single experiment, no matter how thorough, can answer all questions about the effects of a particular treatment for conditions such as ADHD and learning disabilities.

To illustrate this point, let's consider the question "Does sugar have adverse effects on children's behavior?" To the uninitiated, the solution might seem straightforward: compare the behavior of children before and after they receive a "dose" of sugar, and then draw conclusions about the effects of sugar on children's behavior. On closer inspection, however, we find that several questions must be resolved before we can embark on this project. What kinds of children should we study, for example? Should we look at average children in the general population—"the boy next door"? Or should we study only children with ADHD? Or, as some investigators have done, should we compare the two groups? Maybe we should study only those children who have been identified by parents as "sugar responders," as some have done. But what about age range? Since some researchers have suggested that younger and older children differ in their response to sugar, we must decide whether to study toddlers or elementary school children. Of course, it would be nice to include several age groups, but it's not an easy task to locate parents who are willing to allow their children to participate in research projects.

After identifying our target subjects, we must decide which behaviors we should observe and measure. We could observe children from behind one-way mirrors in a laboratory, using measures of attention, activity, aggression, and so on. Or, since we are not always certain how behavior in the laboratory relates to behavior in the real world, we could choose the more ambitious route of observing our subjects in real-life settings, such as in the classroom or on the playground. Keep in mind, however, that it costs a great deal of time and money to hire and train research assistants to serve as observers, so budgetary constraints will place limits on our ambition.

Finally, there are decisions about what kind of sugar to use, how to present it, and how much should constitute a test dose. This is tricky because if we use too little, we might overlook some youngsters who are sensitive to sugar only in higher doses. On the other hand, if we use amounts that are much greater than a child might reasonably consume at home, our findings may be clinically meaningless. There are other questions too, such as whether to administer sugar on an empty stomach or after a meal. One expert believes that we are most likely to observe adverse effects of sugar if it is eaten after the child has already consumed a high-carbohydrate meal. Others, however, have suggested that the child should be deprived of all sugar for at least a week before the study.

We could go on and on with this list, but we think it is abundantly clear that no single experiment could provide a final answer to the question "Does sugar have adverse effects on children's behavior?" Only after many careful experiments, painstakingly conducted, would we be able to draw any firm conclusions about the relationship between sugar and children's behavior.

**ALTERNATIVE TREATMENTS:
ANOTHER PATH**

There is another route, quite different from the scientific approach, by which some treatments attract public attention and gain popular acceptance. Although this path is a much shorter one than that followed by legitimate scientists, it is filled with pitfalls.

On this path, new treatment procedures often spring from ideas which are outside of the mainstream of existing medical and scientific knowledge. There may be no logical connection between the proposed treatment and the ailment it is supposed to cure. In some cases—like the treatment approach based on moving the bones in the skull, discussed in Chapter 9—the theory actually flies in the face of common sense.

Claims for the treatment may be overstated and exaggerated. Results may be described as "astonishing," "miraculous," or "an amazing breakthrough." The words "cure," "painless," "natural," "safe," and "guaranteed" are often used in connection with the treatment, while no mention is made of cost or side effects. There may be repeated references to huge numbers of patients who have been successfully treated, and there may even be testimonials from "satisfied customers." (However, there are seldom, if ever, any reports concerning patients who failed to benefit from the treatment.)

Impressive claims may be made, too, concerning the range of ailments and illnesses which can be helped by the particular treatment. We may be told, for example, that Treatment X leads to improvement in a host of completely unrelated ailments, ranging (literally) from hyperactivity to halitosis.

Proponents of such treatments often present themselves as scientists "on the cutting edge." Professional titles like "Doctor" and "Professor" enhance their credibility in the eyes of the public, and they cite scientific references and use impressive medical or pseudomedical terms to describe their ideas. Their image as authority figures is often bolstered by the fact that when they appear on radio and television talk shows, no other experts are present to critique their theories and present alternative views.

All in all, it can be a very convincing performance. But what happens when we look beyond the hype? Often we find that these treatments are billed as proven and effective long before there is any solid research from which such conclusions might be drawn. Experiments may be poorly designed and focus on small numbers of patients with a grab bag of diagnoses. Measurement techniques and statistical methods used to analyze the results are not described, if they are used at all, and single-case "studies" are offered as proof that the treatment works.

We may find, too, that the treatment approach has been publicized only in obscure books or journals which do not require peer review by recognized experts in the field. Often, in fact, the advocate of a particular approach publishes the work himself through a "vanity press" arrangement in which the author pays the costs involved in publication.

It is also not uncommon to find that parent support groups have been formed to advocate the treatment. Although parent support groups have an important role to play in disseminating information about childhood disorders, support groups which form around alternative treatments advocate one, and only one, approach to treatment. These groups play an important role in publicizing and promoting the particular treatment, usually bolstered by stirring testimonials. Unfortunately, as we have seen, enthusiasm is no substitute for evidence.

In fact, what happens when we ask for evidence? Confronted with this demand, proponents of many alternative treatments take refuge by claiming access to "inside" information which has not yet come to the attention of the general professional community. In the face of criticism and questions, they may invoke a conspiracy theory, claiming that drug companies, food manufacturers, and even medical professionals have a vested interest in keeping "the truth" from the public.

**MAKING INFORMED CHOICES**

It would certainly be unfair to conclude that everyone who proposes a new approach to treating children's learning and behavior problems is a charlatan. After all, who would have ever suspected that a treatment as potent as penicillin could be derived from bread mold?

We believe, however, that parents who purchase services for their children must have some guidelines to follow in determining how and where to allocate time, money, effort, and other scarce resources. We propose that the following questions be used as guidelines in deciding whether or not to pursue a particular treatment for ADHD or learning disabilities.

1. Is this theory consistent with existing knowledge in related fields such as anatomy, medicine, psychiatry, psychology, and education?

2. Is the theory consistent with what is specifically known about ADHD and learning disabilities?

3. What is the quality of the scientific evidence which indicates that the treatment is effective?

4. What are the costs involved and what, if any, are the dangers associated with this treatment?

Let's keep this checklist in mind as we examine controversial methods which have been proposed to treat the problems of children with ADHD and learning disabilities.

## Chapter 4

### Effective Treatments for ADHD

Over the years, the array of remedies which have been proposed for ADHD has grown to mind-boggling proportions. The list of medications, potions, and elixirs alone is a lengthy one, ranging from the widely used stimulant drugs to such exotic substances as oil of evening primrose. A host of special diets have been touted as beneficial, including diets free of sugar, dyes, additives, and other substances presumed to cause learning and behavior problems. Various forms of psychotherapy have been tried, such as play therapy and the currently popular family therapy. Behavior modification programs have been widely used in the home and the classroom. Training approaches aimed at remedying presumed underlying weaknesses have employed eye exercises, instruction in self-control and social skills, exercises to improve sensory motor integration, and biofeedback techniques. Environmental manipulations have included removal of fluorescent lights, isolation of children in individual cubicles in the classroom, and the use of "minimal stimulation" classrooms with frosted windows, bare walls, and teachers dressed in drab colors.

Despite the intuitive appeal of many of these remedies, only a few have survived the rigorous test of controlled scientific evaluation. We summarize these approaches in the following pages.

**STIMULANT MEDICATION**

More than fifty years ago, it was discovered that central nervous system stimulants such as amphetamines had the effect of calming restless, hyperactive children and helping them maintain attention and concentration. This discovery was generally ignored for years, but in the 1960s and '70s, the results of many scientific studies confirmed earlier findings. Interest in the use of stimulants was renewed, and Dexedrine (dextroamphetamine) and Ritalin (methylphenidate) came into widespread use for the treatment of ADHD.

In 1977, Dr. Russell Barkley summarized the results of thirty-one studies involving nearly two thousand children treated with stimulant medication.[1] Improvement rates ranged from 73 to 77 percent overall. More recent reviews of stimulant medication effects have reported equally high or higher rates of improvement.[2]

Today, drug treatment is well established as an effective means of helping children and adults with ADHD. Ritalin is the most frequently prescribed medication, followed by Dexedrine. Cylert (magnesium pemoline) is a relative newcomer. It has been used less often because in the past, at least, effects were not obvious for a period of days to weeks. Recent research, however, suggests that beneficial effects can be obtained more quickly, and there are many who believe that this medication, because it is long-acting, offers advantages in sustained control of symptoms.[3]

*How Do Stimulants Work and What Do They Do?*

Stimulant medication does not simply sedate the ADHD child. Instead, it helps him focus his attention, control his impulsive responses, and regulate his activity level. The exact mechanism of action is not yet known, but all the evidence points to an effect on the neurotransmitters, the chemical messengers in the brain. This means that stimulant medication does not just mask the symptoms of ADHD, as some believe. Instead, it corrects a biochemical condition which interferes with attention and impulse control and, in so doing, acts directly on the cause of the problem.

The very positive and oftentimes dramatic effects of stimulant medication on the behavior of youngsters with ADHD were succinctly described in 1986 by Drs. Keith Conners and Karen Wells, then at Children's Hospital National Medical Center in Washington, D.C.

> Without doubt, the most single striking phenomenon of hyperkinetic children is their response to stimulant drugs. The effect is both immediate and obvious. Often within the first hour after treatment, a perceptible change in handwriting, talking, motility, attending, planfulness and perception may be observed. Classroom teachers may notice improvement in deportment and academic productivity after a single dose. Parents will frequently report a marked reduction in troublesome sibling interactions, inappropriate activity, and non-compliance. Even peers can identify the calmer, more organizing cooperative behavior of stimulant treated children.[4]

### Are There Side Effects or Dangers?

It is clear that there is a substantial body of evidence supporting the important role of stimulant medication in the management of ADHD. Findings from many carefully conducted studies also indicate that stimulant medication, properly employed, is generally quite safe and that side effects are minimal. As long as a decade ago, Dr. Judith Rapoport, Chief of the Child Psychiatry Branch at the National Institute of Mental Health, summed up the evidence as follows: "The data are very good that stimulant drugs are one of the mainstays of treatment ... [for ADHD], Although there are individual cases of overuse or misuse, properly used stimulant drugs can be good treatment."[5]

Yet many parents are reluctant to consider medication in their child's treatment because they have been warned about the dangers of stimulant medication. In fact, it is probably safe to say that myths and misinformation are more commonly encountered around the topic of stimulant medication than around any other aspect of ADHD.

Confusion and conflicting opinions about stimulant medication can be traced to several sources. Misdiagnosis or incomplete diagnosis of the child's problem appears to be a major reason that stimulants have produced unsatisfactory results in some cases. For ADHD children who suffer from coexisting conditions such as depression and anxiety disorders, stimulant medication alone may not be helpful. In fact, it may actually compound problems when a coexisting disorder is present.

In other cases, parents and physicians may mistakenly conclude that certain kinds of problems are due to medication when in reality they are preexisting problems which have gone unnoticed or unremarked upon until medication has been introduced. In fact, careful examination of children on a placebo and on Ritalin indicates that so-called "side effects" such as irritability and excessive staring are essentially the same under both conditions.[6]

Finally, a great deal of the current confusion about stimulant medication can be traced directly to a deliberate campaign of misinformation carried out by an organization known as the Citizens Commission on Human Rights. Despite the organization's impressive title, it is actually funded by the Church of Scientology, a cult described in a *Time* magazine cover story as "The Cult of Greed and Power."[7] The Citizens Commission on Human Rights, which *Time* described as a group "at war with psychiatry, its primary competitor," launched a campaign of distortions, exaggerations, and outright lies about Ritalin in the treatment of ADHD children. Among the unsubstantiated allegations made by this group were the claims that Ritalin is addictive, that its use increases the risk of later drug abuse, and that Ritalin turns children into "zombies."

*Table 4: Myths and Facts About Stimulant Medication*

| Myth | Fact |
| --- | --- |
| Children treated with stimulant medication become addicted. | There is no evidence that treatment with stimulant medication leads to dependence or addiction in ADHD individuals. |
| Stimulant medication stunts growth. | Stimulant medication has minimal effect on ultimate adult height and weight. |
| Stimulant medication turns a child into a "zombie." | Sedation and personality change are not typical side effects of stimulant medication. |
| Stimulant medication is not effective with adolescents. | Treatment with stimulant medication continues to be helpful during teen and adult years. |
| Stimulant medication causes Tourette's syndrome. | There is no evidence that stimulant medication causes Tourette's syndrome. |

Before we examine these myths and other misconceptions about stimulant medication, it is important to note that such treatment can result in some mild side effects. In an evaluation of 110 studies, which included more than forty-two hundred children treated with stimulant medication,[8] primary side effects reported were insomnia, loss of appetite, and weight loss. Other mild but less common side effects included sadness, depression, fearfulness, social withdrawal, sleepiness, headaches, nail biting, and stomach upset. All side effects were generally short-term and the majority disappeared with a reduction in drug dosage. All were considered acceptable in light of clinical improvement.

Now that we have the facts, let's examine the myths about stimulant medication.

**Myth Children Treated with Stimulant Medication Become Addicted.**

**Fact There Is No Evidence That Treatment with Stimulant Medication Leads to Dependence or Addiction in ADHD Individuals.**

Long-term studies have *not* found addiction to, or abuse of, stimulant medication to be a problem for ADHD children and adolescents treated with stimulants. In some cases, children do develop tolerance (the need for increased doses), but this is rare and can usually be managed by switching to a different stimulant or another type of medication, such as an antidepressant.

There is also no evidence that children treated with stimulants have a greater likelihood of illegal drug abuse in later years. In fact, a number of studies have found that ADHD children treated with stimulants were actually less likely to abuse drugs and alcohol in adolescence than those who had not received treatment with stimulants.

Finally, there is no indication that withdrawal from stimulant medication poses the risk of suicide or depression, as some opponents of medication have alleged. This allegation is particularly nonsensical, since individuals treated with stimulants "withdraw" from medication without mishap or discomfort on a daily basis when the last dose of the day wears off.

**Myth Stimulant Medication Stunts Growth.**

**Fact Stimulant Medication Has Minimal Effects on Ultimate Adult Height and Weight.**

Several authorities, including a panel appointed by the U.S. Food and Drug

Administration, have examined this question. They have concluded that although there may be some suppression of growth during the first year or two of treatment, this is a transient problem. Children seem to "catch up" by the second or third year, and any ultimate effects on adult height appear to be minimal.[9]

**Myth Stimulant Medication Turns a Child into a "Zombie."**

**Fact Sedation and Personality Change Are Not Typical Side Effects of Stimulant Medication.**

If medication is used properly, the child should not appear sleepy or "druggy," nor should he complain of feeling tired or sad or "weird." These symptoms may appear when the dose is too high or when a coexisting condition such as a mood disorder has not been properly identified and treated. When the coexisting condition is diagnosed and treated, stimulant medication is then often safely and effectively used in combination with other medications.

**Myth Stimulant Medication Is Not Effective with Adolescents.**

**Fact Treatment with Stimulant Medication Continues to Be Helpful During Teen and Adult Years.**

Convincing evidence[10] indicates that ADHD youngsters continue to benefit from stimulant medication during adolescence and as adults. Despite increased body mass, the amount of medication per dose usually remains the same from late childhood through the adult years.

**Myth Stimulant Medication Causes Tourette's Syndrome.**

**Fact There Is No Convincing Evidence That Stimulant Medication Causes Tourette's Syndrome.**

The most recent evidence does not support the notion that stimulants can produce Tourette's syndrome, a neurological condition characterized by multiple, persistent motor and vocal tics. More than half of children with Tourette's syndrome also have ADHD, which appears months or even years before the onset of tics. Treatment with stimulant medication may "uncover" tics which would have emerged later in the natural course of the syndrome. In the past, a history of tics and the emergence of tics with stimulant medication were considered contraindications to the use of stimulants. It now appears that while some youngsters with Tourette's syndrome cannot tolerate stimulant medication, there are many in whom tics are not worsened by stimulants. There is even some recent research which indicates that, in some children, treatment with stimulant medication actually appears to reduce tics.[11]

**ARE OTHER MEDICATIONS HELPFUL?**

*Tricyclic Antidepressants*

In addition to stimulant medications, a wide variety of drugs have been tried in the treatment of ADHD. Among them, the most carefully studied have been the tricyclic antidepressants, so called because of their chemical structure. Several controlled studies have shown that the tricyclics imipramine and desipramine can produce improvement in up to three quarters of ADHD individuals studied. Improvements in behavior are generally more prominent than improvements in attention (at least as measured by laboratory tasks), and it is thought that the tricyclics work by improving mood, impulsivity, and frustration tolerance.

At lower doses, side effects are not usually a problem with the tricyclics, but at doses higher than 100 milligrams or so, some children may have dry mouth, constipation, and/or drowsiness. Desipramine appears less likely than imipramine to produce these side effects.

Certain precautions must be observed when tricyclics are used to treat ADHD. Like other medications, they should be kept beyond the reach of younger children, because an overdose can be fatal. In children taking tricyclics, the electrocardiogram (EKG) should be monitored regularly by a physician. Finally, if medication is discontinued, it should be withdrawn gradually to avoid the possibility of uncomfortable flulike symptoms, which can occur if this medication is abruptly discontinued.

The tricyclics appear to be a good second line of medication for ADHD children who do not benefit from stimulants or who experience troublesome side effects when on stimulants. In children who have both ADHD and a mood or anxiety disorder, the tricyclic antidepressants should probably be considered the drug of choice.

Clinical experience suggests that there is also a subgroup of children with ADHD and coexisting mood or anxiety disorders who derive the greatest benefit from a combined regimen of stimulant medication and tricyclic antidepressants. Although there are no controlled studies at this time, this approach appears particularly promising. However, until better guidelines have been established, it is an approach which should be undertaken only by a professional who is experienced in the use of psychotropic medications with children.

*Clonidine*

The blood pressure medication clonidine (Catapres) appears to be a promising new treatment for some individuals with ADHD. This medication, which has been used for more than two decades to treat high blood pressure, has been shown to reduce the high level of arousal in ADHD children who are severely overactive, aggressive, and explosive. Dr. Robert Hunt, a psychiatrist at Vanderbilt University Medical School, pioneered controlled research on the use of clonidine with ADHD children. According to Dr. Hunt, "The most responsive ADHD children appear to have an early onset, to be extremely energetic, and often exhibit associated oppositional or conduct disorder."[12] In this group of children, clonidine improves frustration tolerance, which in turn leads to increases in on-task behavior, better learning and effort, and greater cooperativeness.

However, while clonidine reduces arousal, it does not improve distractibility. For youngsters who are both highly aroused and very distractible, Dr. Hunt has found a combined regimen of clonidine and Ritalin to be most helpful. When both drugs were used in combination, Dr. Hunt found that the amount of Ritalin needed could be reduced considerably and, further, that side effects of both medications were reduced.

Clonidine certainly appears to be a promising treatment for a subgroup of youngsters affected by ADHD. The most common short-term side effect is drowsiness, which is usually short-lived (and can actually be a benefit when it is given at bedtime to children who are highly aroused and who would otherwise have difficulty falling asleep). In a small percentage of children, depression may occur, especially if the child or family member has a history of depression. However, children have been treated for as long as five years without developing long-term side effects.[13]

For a child treated with clonidine, it usually takes about two weeks to see any improvement and up to three months to see maximal improvement, since the medication is started at low doses and only gradually increased. As with tricyclics, clonidine should never be discontinued abruptly but should be carefully tapered off under the close supervision of a doctor.

**BEHAVIOR MANAGEMENT AND ENVIRONMENTAL ENGINEERING**

The results of countless studies support the use of behavior management/behavior modification techniques to help the ADHD youngster function optimally at home and in school. Since many excellent books for parents, teachers, and mental health professionals provide detailed explanations and examples of behavior modification methods, we will give only a brief overview, highlighting the most important features of this approach. For more detailed material, see the Addenda.

*What Is Behavior Modification and How Does It Work?*

Behavior modification is based on the idea that specific behaviors are learned because they produce specific effects, or consequences. In general, positive consequences—those which are enjoyable or rewarding—tend to strengthen the behavior, making it more likely that it will occur again. On the other hand, negative consequences— those which are unpleasant or painful— weaken the behavior, making it less likely that it will occur again.

Consequences need not be dramatic in order to be effective. In fact, some social consequences such as praise or even a hug or smile (or frown) can be surprisingly effective in strengthening or weakening behavior. Timing, however, is critical: behavior is affected most strongly by consequences which immediately follow the behavior. Delayed consequences are less effective in bringing about changes in behavior, especially with ADHD children who have difficulty delaying gratification.

**Using Consequences to Change Behavior.** Although we tend to think first of negative, or punishing, consequences when we think about improving child behavior, positive consequences are far more potent tools in bringing about behavior change. Positive consequences, also called "reinforcers," do not have to be elaborate or expensive. Many parents have had good results just by incorporating into a behavior management program the everyday activities children take for granted, like watching television, playing computer games, or playing with friends. Just be sure to be generous with positive consequences: deliver them frequently and reward small steps toward improvement.

Since ADHD children have a "bias toward novelty," they tend to tire of things and become bored more quickly than other children. This means that you can't count on using the same reinforcers over a long period of time or they will cease to be effective. Obviously, then, the effective use of positive consequences demands considerable ingenuity and creativity on the part of parents, but this is not necessarily a drawback. Many parents—once they get into the spirit of things—actually find this both challenging and enjoyable.

Negative consequences are tempting to use because they often bring about immediate, if temporary, changes in behavior. However, since punishment can lead to power plays and ill feelings in the family, it's a good idea to use it judiciously. *Time out,* which involves isolating the child for a few minutes following misbehavior, is a mild but surprisingly effective way in which to deliver negative consequences. Psychologist Tom Phelan's modification of this technique, which makes it even more effective, consists of verbal warnings in the form of "counting the child out."[14] *Response-cost* approaches, in which the child starts out with a certain number of points, minutes of free time, or what have you and is fined for each infraction, are also very effective with ADHD youngsters.

If you decide to undertake a behavior modification program with your child, remember to keep it as simple as possible. Complicated point programs may work well in an institutional setting, but they require more time and effort than the average family can afford over the long haul. Since behavior modification is actually a very sophisticated technology, it's also a good idea to consult a mental health professional with special expertise in the area to maximize the likelihood of success. Parent-training programs, designed to teach parents how to use behavior modification techniques, have been shown to be at least moderately effective in helping parents manage and change difficult behavior in their ADHD children.[15]

**Behavior Modification in the Classroom.** Numerous well-conducted studies attest to the efficacy of behavior modification methods to improve classroom behavior and academic productivity.[16] Although the power of positive consequences for changing behavior has been documented in countless studies, surveys continue to show that teachers employ criticism and negative consequences much more frequently than they make use of praise and positive consequences. This is especially unfortunate, since we know that increases in praise, approval, and positive consequences bring about improved behavior in *all* children in a classroom, not just in those who are the direct recipients of positive consequences.

The response-cost procedure developed by Dr. Mark Rapport is an excellent way in which to combine frequent positive consequences for appropriate behavior in the classroom with mild negative consequences for inappropriate behavior. Dr. Rapport has developed an automated system which awards the child a point every sixty seconds as long as he remains on-task. If he wanders off-task, the teacher uses a remote-control device to deduct a point and activate a warning light. Research supports the effectiveness of this system in increasing appropriate behavior, and teachers report that it is quite simple to use.[17] We have also used this system at home to help youngsters stay on-task while doing homework.

An alternative to teacher monitoring of on-task behavior is to teach ADHD children to monitor their own attention and concentration. A good way to teach self-monitoring is to provide children with "concentration tapes," audiotapes on which a beep sounds randomly every thirty to sixty seconds. Each time the child hears the beep, he checks to be sure he is concentrating on his work instead of daydreaming or bugging his neighbor. This approach has been evaluated in several studies and has been shown to be quite helpful.[18] Since a version is now commercially available,[19] parents can also use this approach to help youngsters self-monitor their concentration while doing homework.

*Other Accommodations in the Classroom*

The ideal classroom for the ADHD child is one which is highly structured and well organized, with clear rules and a predictable schedule. Expectations must be adjusted to meet the child's skill level, and academic material should be matched to the child's ability. At Purdue University, Dr. Sydney Zentall has found that ADHD youngsters perform better if they can be active participants in learning tasks, so she suggests that tasks for these children include an active component like turning over flash cards.[20] Because these children have such a high need for novelty, Dr. Zentall has also found it helpful to present brief assignments and to vary the way in which the material is presented.

Other helpful classroom accommodations for children with ADHD include preferential seating (placing the child's desk near the teacher and away from windows or high-traffic areas) and allowing extra time on tests, since the ADHD child often works slowly. Because ADHD children usually have problems organizing themselves, their belongings, and their work-space, they can benefit from help in keeping their notebooks and desks orderly and uncluttered. They can also benefit enormously from a daily homework journal or assignment pad, particularly if both teachers and parents are required to initial the journal daily, attesting to the fact that the homework has been assigned, completed, and turned in.*

Since the school setting is often the one in which ADHD children encounter the greatest amount of difficulty, it is imperative that these youngsters receive the support they need to help them function well in the classroom. It is also the law. In September 1991, the United States Department of Education issued a policy memorandum which stated, in part:

> Children with ADD should be classified as eligible for services under the "other health impaired" category in instances where the ADD is a chronic or acute health problem that results in limited alertness, which adversely affects educational performance.[21]

This does not mean that every child with ADHD requires special services and accommodations in school. Many, in fact, do not. However, for ADHD youngsters who do need such services, federal law requires that they be provided.

---

* Two publications which offer a wealth of useful information about helping the ADHD child in the classroom are The ADD Hyperactivity Handbook for Schools and the CH.A.D.D. Educator's Manual (see Addenda).

# Chapter 5

### Effective Treatments for Learning Disabilities

Although the plight of children with learning disabilities has only recently received widespread attention, interest in the subject has a long history. In fact, the professional literature dates back to 1877, when A. Kussmaul coined the term "word-blindness" to describe an inability to read in spite of normal vision.

Despite a huge body of literature devoted to learning disabilities, there is surprisingly little in the way of solid information on the most effective ways to treat learning-disabled children. In fact, when Dr. Doris Johnson summarized the research on learning disabilities for the 1987 National Conference on Learning Disabilities, she found that out of four hundred studies, a mere 5 percent dealt with treatment.[1]

Of this small number, an even smaller number could be considered acceptable by scientific standards. When Dr. William Feldman reviewed the research on treatment of learning disabilities in 1990 for his book *Learning Disabilities: A Review of Available Treatments*,[2] more than half the articles he located through an exhaustive search had little or no value as scientific evidence. Most were position papers describing a particular theory or case studies involving only one or two learning-disabled children.

The paucity of solid research concerning the treatment of learning disabilities is, in many ways, understandable. Such research is more expensive and much more time-consuming than most people realize. In order to design and carry out scientifically acceptable research, it is also necessary to have at least one member of the study team who has been thoroughly trained in research methodology, statistics, and the like. Teachers and other professionals interested in working with learning-impaired children usually do not receive such training and so are ill-equipped to undertake research projects.

This state of affairs is frustrating and disappointing, particularly to parents. After they have spent a great deal of money to have their child's learning problems evaluated and assessed, it is not unreasonable for them to expect recommendations for remedial procedures of proven effectiveness. Sadly, this is not always the case.

It is not that there has been a dearth of programs put forth to treat learning disabilities—not at all! Proposed remediation programs have included everything from visual-motor training as a means of improving reading to teaching children how to crawl, on the theory that this would improve communication between the right and left sides of the brain. Very few of these programs, however, have ever been subjected to close scientific scrutiny, and when they have been, most have been found ineffective.

In the following sections, we will describe the approaches that have stood up to scientific evaluation. These approaches fall into two main categories: 1) those which employ medication to enhance central nervous system functioning; and 2) those which are educational in nature.

## MEDICATION FOR LEARNING DISABILITIES

*Stimulant Medication*

Regardless of whether they have actual learning disabilities, children with ADHD usually have problems with academic performance. Since this is the case, many studies assessing the effects of stimulant medication have examined the effects on academic performance, as well as on hyperactivity and impulsivity. These studies have clearly demonstrated that stimulant medication can result in considerable improvement in academic performance, as we will discuss below.

However, there is also a group of youngsters with learning problems who do not seem to have coexisting problems with attention and impulse control. When these children are given stimulant medication, the results are not nearly as clear-cut. Therefore, we will consider this group separately.

**Children with Learning and Attention Problems.** Early on, when researchers examined the effects of stimulant medication on children in whom both learning and attention problems were apparent, the results did not appear promising. However, as researchers refined their methods and measures, it soon became apparent that ADHD children treated with stimulant medication often showed impressive gains in both work output and accuracy in the areas of spelling, reading, and arithmetic. The amount of improvement observed was quite substantial, ranging from 25 to 40 percent. In one study, for example, medication resulted in a 30 percent increase in the number of arithmetic problems completed, with no loss in accuracy.[3] In another study, researchers reported a 25 percent improvement in spelling tasks as a result of medication.[4]

A heated debate arose among behavioral scientists concerning the reasons underlying these clear-cut improvements: Were they due simply to the fact that the youngsters settled down, stopped wandering around the room, and devoted their attention to their academic work? Or was it the case that stimulant medication was exerting a more direct effect on the brain processes and mechanisms involved in learning?

At this time, the answer seems to be that stimulant medication works at both levels. It is not surprising that researchers have found a strong relationship between improvements in behavior and improvements in academic performance following medication: it makes sense that children are more likely to produce complete, accurate work products when they are able to remain seated and focus on the task at hand. However, stimulant medication also seems to have a beneficial effect on the way in which the central nervous system "processes" information. In reading tasks, specifically, this effect is seen in improved word-finding abilities rather than in improved phonicskills.[5]

The effects of stimulants on central processing mechanisms may account for the fact that stimulants also improve the academic performance of youngsters who have attentional problems without behavioral difficulties (called "Attention Deficit Disorder without Hyperactivity" in DSM III and "Undifferentiated Attention Deficit Disorder" in DSM III-R). These children are often disorganized, forgetful, daydreamy, lethargic, and generally rather sluggish in responding to tasks. They seem to process information slowly and they have difficulty retrieving information from memory. In addition to beneficial effects on attention, stimulant medication seems to improve processing in these children. Interestingly, these youngsters seem to respond to lower doses of medication than are usually required to help children who are also impulsive and hyperactive.[6]

In spite of these documented improvements, it is clear that stimulant medication alone is not always sufficient to help learning-impaired youngsters with attentional problems who have fallen far behind their classmates. Common sense dictates that these children receive specific remedial help to enable them to make up for lost time. Research is quite clear in showing that for youngsters with both ADHD and reading disorders, the greatest improvements in reading result when the children are treated with a combination of stimulant medication and remedial teaching.[7]

**Children Without Attentional Problems**. When we ask "Is stimulant medication helpful to learning-impaired children who do *not* have obvious accompanying attentional problems?" we are on less solid ground in terms of scientific evidence. We have only a few studies in which dyslexic children without accompanying attentional problems have been studied, so the available evidence is very scanty. Studies conducted by psychologist Rachel Gittelman at Columbia University[8] seem to indicate that the contribution of stimulant medication to improved reading skills in these children is minimal.

**EDUCATIONAL APPROACHES**

Until recently, the most popular approaches to remediation of learning disabilities were those which used *indirect* remedial methods; that is, methods which focus on presumed underlying perceptual problems or motivational problems. Among these approaches, the best known have concentrated on perceptual problems, like the well-known Frostig Program, which involves training in discriminating various patterns, forms, and sounds. These approaches, however, have not stood up to scientific scrutiny. They have been replaced by more direct approaches which focus on teaching and practicing the specific skills required for the task at hand.

*Reading Remediation Methods*

Many educators have argued quite persuasively that the most logical way to teach reading to all children—with or without learning disabilities—is to provide direct and intensive training in reading skills. This, in fact, is the procedure which tutors and reading teachers have relied on for many years.

There are also a number of special programs which have been specifically designed to teach letter-sound relations and sound blending. Among the better known are the Orton-Gillingham, the Slingerland, and the DISTAR approaches. Other programs, such as the Lindamood Auditory Discrimination in Depth program, teach phoneme-awareness skills. Still other programs offer specific treatment strategies based on the child's individual profile of strengths and weaknesses.

With the existence of all these programs, one might assume there is solid evidence that such approaches are helpful to reading-disabled children. Once again, however, we are disappointed to find that this is not the case.

There are some clinical studies exploring the effectiveness of phonological awareness training which suggest that it is useful with severely dyslexic children.[9] To date, however, there has been only a single well-controlled study of reading remediation procedures with reading-disabled youngsters.

This study,[10] conducted at Columbia University, used an intensive phonetic teaching program, as well as rewards to motivate children to participate actively. After fifty-four sessions, provided over an eighteen-week period, reading-disabled children showed clear-cut gains in reading skills which were maintained over time. Although these gains were impressive, the children were still not reading at grade level at the end of the study. However, an eighteen-week program can hardly be expected to fully remediate the reading problems of children who are, as these youngsters were, at least two years below grade level in their reading skills.

On a much more encouraging note, there are some excellent studies which clearly demonstrate the value of providing intensive phonics training to preschool children who are "at risk" to become learning-disabled. These preventive studies, conducted by Dr. Rebecca Felton and her associates at Bowman Gray University in North Carolina,[11] and Dr. Pat Lindamood in California,[12] among others, indicate that early intervention methods can be very helpful to children who would otherwise be likely to encounter significant learning problems.

*Strategies Training*

Some professionals in the field of learning disabilities have speculated that learning-disabled children suffer from a lack of learning strategies; that is, they are essentially rather passive learners who do not know how to tackle learning situations in an efficient, effective manner. Thus, these children have difficulty devising plans of action which allow them to gather information in a systematic fashion.

If this is in fact the case, we should be able to help learning-disabled children by teaching them very specific strategies to improve the way in which they approach new tasks, break down and memorize new information, and organize it when they are tested on it. Researchers have explored this approach and, in the process, have come up with some good ways to help learning-disabled children "learn how to learn."

What kinds of strategies have they found to be most helpful? Foremost among them are techniques aimed at helping students improve their ability to memorize. Mnemonic (the "m" is silent in this apparently impossible word) techniques consist of formulas and other aids to memory. For example, children might be taught to use visual images, rhymes, and jingles to link specific bits of information together.

These strategies have been shown to yield consistent improvement in recall. In one well-controlled investigation,[13] for example, learning-disabled adolescents were given mnemonic strategy training and memory-jogging illustrations to help them learn science facts. Results were quite impressive: students with whom these techniques were used scored 93 percent on the actual science test, while those not trained with this approach scored only 55 percent.

One very simple teaching strategy that has been found effective with learning-disabled children is the so-called "write-say" method. This approach involves having the student rewrite incorrectly spelled words several times while simultaneously spelling the word aloud. The write-say method, which provides the child with immediate feedback in both the visual and auditory channels, has been shown to enhance the spelling accuracy of learning-disabled children in a brief period of time.[14] A variant of this procedure has also been used successfully to teach multiplication tables to learning-disabled children.[15]

Researchers have also explored other kinds of strategies to improve different areas of academic performance. One group of investigators taught learning-disabled children specific strategies to use when taking tests, with good results.[16] Other investigators have demonstrated beneficial effects when teaching learning-impaired children to scan the material, pay close attention to its important aspects, talk themselves through various steps in problem solving, and monitor their own performance. These cognitive strategies have been used successfully to improve performance in reading and arithmetic.[17,18]

*Peer Tutoring*

In peer tutoring, as the term implies, other children in the same class or school serve as tutors for children who have learning problems. It is not that some children are "smarter" than others; rather, in a group of children, different kinds of information will be mastered at various rates by the individuals in the group. Children who have mastered a particular skill or concept can help others who have not yet achieved mastery. In the process of serving as tutors, their own learning is also enhanced.

The benefits of this approach have long been recognized in medical education. Peer tutoring plays an important role as students learn and master complicated medical procedures through the "see one, do one, teach one" method.

In the elementary school classroom, a small but convincing body of research indicates that learning-impaired children can benefit from working cooperatively with their non-learning-disabled peers to improve math and spelling skills. These studies have also clearly demonstrated that peer tutoring results in mutual benefits to tutor and tutee alike and that gains are maintained over time.[19]

Peer tutoring also appears to increase social interaction with, and acceptance of, learning-disabled children by their peers. Since children with learning problems are often not well liked or tolerated by other children, such increased acceptance is certainly an important by-product of this approach.

Based on these findings, it is astonishing that peer tutoring has not been more widely utilized. By all indications, it is an effective and inexpensive way to help learning-disabled children, while at the same time benefiting the non-learning-disabled youngsters who participate.

*Computers*

Using computers to help learning-disabled children improve their academic skills has a great deal of intuitive appeal. Computers should be excellent "teachers" for these children because they repeat a task as many times as necessary without becoming impatient, and they provide immediate feedback. Computers also have an inherent appeal to most children—so much so, in fact, that in many schools where children have access to computers, loss of computer time is a potent penalty for unacceptable behavior. Research supports informal observations that children appear highly motivated when using a computer and that they stay on-task for long periods of time.

Results of early studies on the use of computers to help learning-impaired children were equivocal. Recently, however, well-controlled studies have shown that computer programs designed to improve phonics skills in reading-disabled children can produce impressive results. At Florida State University, for example, Dr. Joseph Torgeson demonstrated substantial gains in decoding skills in a group of dyslexic children as a result of a ten-week program which involved just fifteen minutes a day for five days a week.[20]

In Colorado, Drs. Richard Olson and Barbara Wise[21] have used computer-assisted instruction methods with young children at high risk for learning disabilities. The results of their research offer the promise that through early intervention many children who would otherwise struggle and fall behind in reading can go on to become normal readers.

# SECTION III
## Out of the Mainstream: Controversial Treatments for Learning and Attention Problems

## Chapter 6

### Pills and Potions

Since Ponce de Leon hacked his way through the swamps of Florida in search of the mythical Fountain of Youth, Americans have devoted vast amounts of money, energy, and talent to the quest for medicines to treat illness and enhance health and well-being. In many ways, the results have been little short of miraculous. Drugs like antibiotics and insulin have saved countless lives and alleviated much suffering. In the held of psychiatry, antidepressants and other drugs have freed thousands from confinement in institutions and from the inner torment of mental illness.

In Chapter 4, we discussed the benefits of medications such as the stimulants and the tricyclic antidepressants. Are there other substances which might also help children with learning and behavior problems?

**THE ORTHOMOLECULAR APPROACH: MEGAVITAMINS AND MINERAL SUPPLEMENTS**

The use of very high ("mega") doses of vitamins and mineral supplements to treat mental disorders is based on the precepts of orthomolecular psychiatry. This approach advocates treating mental disorders by providing an "optimum molecular environment for the mind."[1] According to this theory, some people have a genetic abnormality which results in increased requirements for specific substances, such as vitamins and minerals, which are normally present in the body. When these higher-than-normal requirements are not met, illness results.

*Vitamin Therapy*

In the 1950s and '60s, the use of massive vitamin doses was applied to the treatment of schizophrenia, a severe form of mental illness, by Drs. Abram Hoffer and Humphry Osmond.[2] Their initial regimen consisted of enormous doses of nicotinic acid or nicotinamide (vitamin $B_3$), to which they later added vitamin C and pyridoxine.

This approach to treating mental illness gained prominence when it was supported by Nobel Prize-winning chemist Linus Pauling. In fact, it was Pauling who coined the term "orthomolecular psychiatry." In the early 1970s, Dr. Allan Cott published several papers in which he claimed that treating hyperactive and learning-disabled children with megavitamins could result in decreased hyperactivity and improvements in attention and concentration.[3] Dr. Cott also claimed that large doses of minerals and hypoglycemic diets were of benefit to behaviorally disordered children.

**The Evidence.** Because vitamins are virtually synonymous with good health, using them to treat learning and behavior disorders has intuitive appeal. The fact that they are a "natural" substance lends them an aura of safety which is reassuring to many people.

The theory itself seems reasonable. We know that although the body cannot manufacture vitamins, they are necessary for normal metabolism, growth, and development. We know, too, that vitamin deficiencies can cause an array of serious diseases. Lack of vitamin D, for example, results in abnormal bone growth and malformed teeth, while vitamin C deficiency can cause scurvy, a condition in which the joints ache, the gums bleed, and teeth loosen and fall out. Lack of the B vitamin niacin can result in pellagra, with physical symptoms such as diarrhea, nausea, and vomiting, and mental symptoms such as confusion, disorientation, and memory impairment. Since vitamin deficiencies can cause such dramatic symptoms, it does not seem so far-fetched to speculate that vitamin deficiencies could also result in more subtle symptoms like learning and behavior disorders.

In spite of the intuitive appeal of this approach, there is *no* solid scientific evidence which supports it. Dr. Cott's claims are based only on his reported clinical experience, and he offers no hard data to support his claims.

Only three studies have reported beneficial effects of megavitamin therapy in children with learning or behavior problems.

- In one,[4] a group of sixteen learning-disabled children treated with megavitamins made more gains in reading and IQ scores than a group treated only with a diet low in sugar and "toxic metals." However, this study did not employ random group assignment or double-blind procedures.
- In a study of one hundred hyperactive children,[5] twenty-four of them improved on vitamins and relapsed on a placebo, but this was an open (nonblind) trial, so the placebo effect cannot be ruled out.
- A third study,[6] employing a regimen of megavitamins and other supplements, thyroid medication, and a sugar-restricted diet, reportedly produced substantial gains in IQ scores in twenty-two mentally retarded children. However, these findings were not corroborated by scores obtained by an independent psychologist, nor were blind procedures used throughout the entire study.

On the negative side, three studies which did employ double-blind and placebo controls failed to find any beneficial effects of megavitamin therapy with hyperactive or learning-disabled children.[7,8,9] The importance of using double-blind procedures is nicely illustrated in one of these studies, conducted by Dr. Robert Haslam and his associates at the University of Calgary.

In this carefully conducted study, forty-one ADHD children were treated with megavitamins in an open (nonblind) manner for three months. Twelve children who demonstrated improvement on parent and teacher ratings were then entered into the second phase of the study, which consisted of two six-week periods on megavitamins and two six-week periods off megavitamins. During this twenty-four-week period, when participants and researchers alike were kept blind as to treatments, four of the children actually exhibited *more* disruptive behavior on megavitamins than when they received a placebo.

What about side effects? The studies cited above remind us that even "natural" substances, when administered in unnatural doses, can prove harmful. In three of them, reported side effects included nausea, loss of appetite, abdominal pain, rashes, flushing, zinc deficiency, and calcium loss. In one of these studies, 42 percent of the children had abnormal liver tests while receiving megavitamins.

**Conclusions.** As long ago as 1973, a task force appointed by the American Psychiatric Association reviewed the available evidence and concluded that use of megavitamins to treat psychiatric, behavioral, and learning problems was not justified. Three years later, the American Academy of Pediatrics Committee on Nutrition specifically stated, "Megavitamin treatment therapy as a treatment for learning disabilities and [other psychiatric conditions] in children ... is not justified on the basis of documented clinical results."[10]

No one disputes the fact that vitamins are necessary for good health, but when used in excessive doses, they can actually be harmful. This is particularly true for those in the fat-soluble group (A, D, E, K). In fact, according to FDA regulations, preparations of vitamins A and D above a certain dose level cannot be obtained without a prescription. Excess vitamin D can lead to loss of appetite, vomiting, weakness, anxiety, depression, abnormal thirst, and changes in kidney function. Too much vitamin A can result in hypervitaminosis A, with symptoms of headaches, fatigue, nausea, diarrhea, and hair loss.

Even water-soluble vitamins are not safe in excess: too much vitamin C, for example, can interfere with the absorption of vitamin $B_{12}$ and may lead to the formation of painful kidney stones. In high doses over a long period of time, nicotinic acid can produce skin rashes and itching, rapid heart rate, liver damage, and increases in blood sugar.

There are medical conditions for which vitamin supplements are indicated. These include pregnancy and nursing, as well as disorders in which vitamins are not properly absorbed by the body. In the absence of these conditions, however, a reasonable diet provides all necessary vitamins.

In summary, there is no evidence which supports the use of very high doses of vitamins to treat learning and behavior problems, but there are documented dangers to this approach. It should not be used in the treatment of children with ADHD or learning disabilities.

Mineral Therapy

Minerals, like vitamins, are necessary for the maintenance of health. At least thirteen minerals have been identified as essential to health, including potassium, sodium, calcium, magnesium, and phosphorus. Others like zinc and copper—so-called "trace elements"—are needed only in tiny amounts.

Proponents of orthomolecular medicine claim that mineral deficiencies can result in learning and behavior problems. They also claim that such deficiencies can be detected by measuring the concentration of certain minerals in the hair and that supplemental treatment with the appropriate minerals will result in improvement in learning and behavior problems.

**The Evidence.** Like the orthomolecular theory of vitamin deficiency, the notion that learning and behavior problems can result from mineral deficiencies has an intuitive appeal and, on the face of it, seems to make sense. We know that minerals are indeed necessary for health and that mineral deficiencies can result in a broad range of problems. Iron, for example, is an essential component of hemoglobin, the oxygen-carrying component of the blood. Iron deficiency results in anemia, which is characterized by pallor, fatigue, headaches, and shortness of breath. Magnesium deficiency, which can occur as a result of alcohol abuse or prolonged treatment with diuretic drugs, can produce anxiety, restlessness, tremors, palpitations, and depression.

This theory, however, is not consistent with what is actually known about mineral deficiencies, which, with the exception of anemia and magnesium deficiency, are quite rare in any population which receives a minimally adequate diet. Nor are there any well-controlled studies which provide support for the theory or for the treatment approach.

Finally, there is good evidence that hair analysis, the technique usually used to detect mineral deficiencies, is not a valid way to measure the levels present in the body. As one expert has pointed out, levels of minerals in hair can be affected by the exposure of hair to the environment, the presence of minerals in some shampoos, hair color, and the rate of hair growth. Therefore, there may be no relationship between levels present in the body and those measured in the hair.

**Conclusions.** Like vitamins, minerals are necessary for normal physical and mental functioning, and like vitamins, they pose dangers when taken in excessive amounts. An excess of iron, for example, can result in nausea, abdominal pain, and liver damage. In excessive amounts, zinc can interfere with the body's ability to absorb iron and copper, in turn resulting in nausea, vomiting, fever, headaches, fatigue, and abdominal pain.

There are documented dangers associated with this approach and no evidence to support its usefulness. Therefore, mineral therapy has no place in the treatment of children with learning or behavior problems.

**ANTI-MOTION-SICKNESS MEDICATION:**
**ADHD AND THE INNER EAR**

One of the more unusual theories about ADHD and learning disabilities has been advanced by Dr. Harold Levinson, a physician who practices in Great Neck, New York.[11]

Dr. Levinson believes that dysfunction in the cerebellar-vestibular system —the inner-ear system—causes a very wide range of problems. His list includes not only ADHD and learning disabilities but speech and language disorders, memory problems, nausea, dizziness, double vision, bedwetting, soiling, migraine headaches, mood swings, nightmares, obsessive compulsive symptoms, anxiety attacks, and low self-esteem.

To understand Dr. Levinson's hypothesis, it is necessary to understand the broad functions of the cerebellar-vestibular (CV) system. One of its components, the *vestibular system,* is located in the inner ear. Within the labyrinth of the inner ear, one type of vestibular receptor responds to the forces of gravity, while a second type responds to the position and movement of the head. The vestibulocochlear nerve carries information from these receptors to the brain, where it is collated with other incoming information by the *cerebellum.* The cerebellum is a part of the brain which plays a very important role in the coordination of voluntary movement. Damage to the cerebellum can result in problems with posture, balance, walking, running, and fine motor skills such as writing, dressing, eating, and smooth tracking movements of the eyes. These two systems, the cerebellum and the vestibular system, together with their complex interconnections, comprise the CV system.

According to Dr. Levinson, the inner ear also regulates the body's energy levels, so a disturbance in this system can produce hyperactivity, impulsivity—even hypo (decreased) activity. Malfunctions in this system can also result in "sensory scrambling," Dr. Levinson's term for a condition in which the brain cannot use the information coming in from the various senses. This, he says, can take the form of difficulty in shutting out distracting sounds; reading problems due to reversals and omissions; specific problems with spelling, arithmetic, and writing; memory problems; and a host of other difficulties.

In his recent book, *Total Concentration,*[12] Dr. Levinson focuses specifically on ADHD and learning disabilities. He claims to have evaluated more than twenty thousand people with ADHD and dyslexia, the majority of whom had problems with balance and coordination. His findings, he states, led him to develop a new classification system for ADHD. According to this system, there are four "primary" types of concentration disorders and one "secondary" type, which he believes results from energy drain resulting from anemia and other medical conditions. Of the four primary types of concentration disorder, he attributes one type to "realistic emotional trauma," a second type to "unconscious neurotic conflicts," and a third type to neurotransmitter dysfunction in the concentration-modulating systems of the brain. However, since the majority of his patients had balance and coordination problems, he concludes that the most common type of concentration disorder reflects a malfunction in the inner ear.

Dr. Levinson also believes that ADHD and learning disabilities reflect the same underlying disorder; that is, individuals with dyslexia also suffer from inner ear-related problems. According to his reasoning, the eye-tracking difficulties observed when dyslexics read are similar to the impairment experienced by normal individuals when reading in a car on a bumpy road or while in a boat on a rough sea. Thus, he concludes that dyslexia can be viewed as a form of dizziness or motion sickness which might respond to treatment with anti-motion-sickness medication.

In fact, Dr. Levinson is best known for his claims that anti-motion-sickness medications like Dramamine are useful in treating the symptoms listed above. Depending on the individual patient, Dr. Levinson also employs a wide array of other medications, including such disparate substances as the potent neuroleptic Mellaril, the tricyclic antidepressants, antihistamines such as Benadryl, and "vitaminlike substances" such as vitamin B complex and gingerroot.

Dr. Levinson includes stimulant medications on this list. In one unpublished study in which he says he investigated the response of one hundred ADHD children to a combination of antihistamines and stimulants, 90 percent of the children responded positively.

Using a combination of various medications, Dr. Levinson also claims to have had success in treating dyslexia. In fact, he states that his treatment has led to the improvement or disappearance of dyslexic symptoms in 75 to 80 percent of the patients he has treated.

### The Evidence

At a minimum, Dr. Levinson's theory is quite inconsistent with anything that is currently known about ADHD, learning disabilities, or the other psychiatric conditions, such as obsessive-compulsive disorder and panic disorder, which he attributes to malfunctions in the inner ear.

It is true that some researchers have reported abnormal eye movements in dyslexics when reading. However, as we discussed in Chapter 2, faulty eye movements appear to be a result of poor reading skills rather than a cause.

It is also true that many ADHD youngsters have problems with motor coordination, especially fine motor coordination. Dr. Levinson's figure of 90 percent, however, is far higher than figures cited by acknowledged experts in the field of ADHD. Other claims made by Dr. Levinson about ADHD—for example, that over 90 percent of ADHD individuals are also learning-disabled and that the incidence of ADHD in the population is over three times as high as current estimates suggest—are similarly inconsistent with research findings.

Most important, there is no body of research literature that supports a link between attentional processes and either the cerebellum or the vestibular system. Anatomically and physiologically, there is no reason to believe that these systems are involved in attention and impulse control in other than the most peripheral ways.

On the other hand, there are compelling reasons to believe that attention and impulse control are regulated in frontal and prefrontal cortical areas of the brain, as we discussed in Chapter 1. Dr. Levinson makes no specific mention of these areas of the brain.

In terms of what is known about the role of specific regions of the central nervous system in conditions such as anxiety disorders and obsessive-compulsive disorder, Dr. Levinson's theory again finds no support. Internationally recognized experts Drs. Thomas Uhde[13] and Judith Rapoport[14] at the National Institute of Mental Health have indeed implicated certain regions of the brain in these difficult and troublesome psychiatric conditions, but their findings do not in any way involve the systems described by Dr. Levinson.

Dr. Levinson states that he has treated more than twenty thousand people with ADHD and that the information he summarizes in his book *Total Concentration* is based on "the largest sample [of ADHD individuals] ever recorded and analyzed." He also refers to a study in which he treated one hundred ADHD children with medication. Does this mean that he is able to back up his claims with findings from well-controlled investigations, the results of which have been published in appropriate scientific journals?

Perhaps it comes as no surprise that this is not the kind of evidence upon which Dr. Levinson relies. Instead, he provides anecdotes in which "scores of suffering and successfully treated people share their amazing insights." Although he has published reports of his work in a refereed journal,[15] the reports consist only of case studies. It is particularly interesting that Dr. Levinson has outlined an acceptable scientific method to evaluate his ideas, but he has not actually used it to put his notions to the test.

In fact, Dr. Levinson cautions prospective patients that they should not expect to read about his theory in "the vast and sometimes perplexing scientific literature." He also warns that people should not expect that their doctor will know of, or understand, his theory, since he believes that "clinical researchers and the medical community at large [have] overlooked the most important piece of the ADD puzzle."

In fact, the scant scientific evidence which does exist concerning Dr.

Levinson's notions fails to support his theory.[16] In a controlled, double-blind study, Dr. Joel Fagan and his associates at the University of Calgary administered meclizine, an anti-motion-sickness medication, to dyslexic children on a short-term and long-term (three-month) basis. Although medication improved eye-movement patterns, it did not lead to improvements in reading skills.

*Conclusions*

Dr. Levinson's theories and methods are outside the mainstream of current practice in ADHD and learning disabilities. In the absence of convincing documentation that this approach is beneficial, it should not be employed in the treatment of ADHD or learning disabilities.

**CANDIDA YEAST AND ADHD**

Yeasts are a type of fungus, a group of plantlike organisms which includes mushrooms and molds. One family of yeasts, known as *Candida albicans*, lives in the human body, especially in the gastrointestinal tract and the vagina. Under normal conditions, their growth in these regions is kept under control by "friendly" bacteria as well as by the action of a strong immune system. However, Candida can multiply and overgrow when friendly bacteria are killed by antibiotics or when the immune system is weakened by illness or other factors. Yeast growth is also encouraged by certain diseases, such as diabetes mellitus, and by hormonal changes caused by pregnancy or by taking birth control pills.

One well-known result of yeast overgrowth is the vaginal yeast infection known as candidiasis. Less commonly, yeast infections can affect the skin, nails, and mouth.

The theory that yeast infections can also cause ADHD has been put forth by Dr. William G. Crook, a pediatrician and allergist who practices in Jackson, Tennessee. According to Dr. Crook, toxins produced by the yeasts circulate through the body and weaken the immune system, making the individual susceptible to a frightening array of infections and illnesses. As Dr. Crook points out in his book *The Yeast Connection*,[17] the list of resulting mental and physical ailments includes ADHD and other psychiatric difficulties, such as suicidal depression, mood swings, and anxiety, as well as hives, psoriasis, headaches, muscle and joint pains, fatigue, infertility, impotence, small breasts, painful intercourse, digestive problems, nasal congestion, insomnia, premenstrual tension, body odor, and bad breath—and this is the short list!

Other than his claim that toxins produced by yeast overgrowth weaken the immune system and "irritate the nervous system," Dr. Crook does not specifically explain how yeast infections result in ADHD. He also does not comment on the origins of learning disabilities, other than to note that many of the hyperactive youngsters he has treated have also had learning disabilities.

He is, however, quite explicit in the treatment plan he outlines for ADHD children, a program which he claims will help over 75 percent of ADHD children. This program, described in Dr. Crook's book *Help for the Hyperactive Child*,[18] includes the following elements:

- A diet low in sugar, additives, and foods to which the child is allergic or sensitive. Because Dr. Crook believes that sugar stimulates yeast growth, he advocates a low-sugar diet. He is also wary of foods which contain artificial flavors, colors, and additives, and he recommends an elimination diet to identify foods to which a child might be allergic or sensitive. An elimination diet involves removing the suspected foods for a period of time and observing behavior changes. Offending foods are then reintroduced and the child is observed to see whether behavior worsens in response.

- A "clean" environment. Like Dr. Doris Rapp, Dr. Crook thinks that many children with learning and behavior problems are sensitive to chemical pollutants and molds in the environment. He suggests that parents try to identify these sensitivities so that offending substances can then be avoided.

- Anticandida therapy. For children who have a history of repeated use of antibiotics, Dr. Crook recommends a course of antifungal medication, such as nystatin. This medication kills yeasts without affecting friendly bacteria.

- Nutritional supplements. Citing the theories of Linus Pauling and other orthomolecular practitioners, Dr. Crook believes that many ADHD children can benefit from supplemental doses of vitamins, minerals, and essential fatty acids.

- An appropriate educational program. For many ADHD and learning-disabled youngsters, small classrooms and tutoring are helpful.

- Consistent discipline and "psychological vitamins" like praise and attention to enhance self-esteem.

*The Evidence*

Criticizing some of Dr. Crook's recommendations would be like attacking motherhood and apple pie. We certainly agree—who would not?—with his advice to limit television viewing, make reasonable rules, and set limits you can enforce, and to spend more "quality time" with your child.

Other aspects of his treatment program are much more controversial, beginning with his notion that the yeast *Candida albicans* is a major cause not only of ADHD but of virtually all ailments to which humans are prey. In his book *The Yeast Connection,* he does add the following disclaimer: "Obviously, Candida isn't 'the cause' of AIDS ... PMS, depression, psoriasis, headache, fatigue, or multiple sclerosis." However, this caveat runs counter to the theme of the other pages of the book.

Is Dr. Crook's theory consistent with existing medical knowledge, in general? While Candida is known to cause infections of the vagina, mouth, and skin, current medical knowledge provides no support for the notion that Candida is a major causative factor in the host of other illnesses listed by Dr. Crook. The existence of a "candidiasis hypersensitivity syndrome" has not been demonstrated, and in 1986, the American Academy of Allergy and Immunology described the condition as "speculative and unproven."[19]

In fact, as far as the illnesses Dr. Crook links to Candida are concerned, he seems to have confused the direction of the cause-effect relationship. In other words, a Candida infection does not cause the illness but simply takes advantage of the body's weakened state to flourish, grow, and produce its own problems and symptoms.

Dr. Crook's theory is also not consistent with current knowledge concerning ADHD. Although he states that "to help the hyperactive child, many pieces need to be put into place," he goes on to describe these pieces as "food allergies, nutritional needs ... appropriate light." None of these approaches have been shown to have merit in treating ADHD.

In lieu of scientific evidence, Dr. Crook provides many pages of anecdotes from his clinical practice, as well as glowing testimonials from other doctors who have used his approach with their patients. Unfortunately, the enthusiasm behind the testimonials cannot in any way substitute for evidence gathered through scientific investigation. As Dr. Crook himself acknowledges in *The Yeast Connection* in a statement addressed to the professional who reads his book:

> [Y]ou may feel that the candida-human illness hypothesis is "speculative" and "unproven" ... [and] ... that double blind and other scientific studies to document this hypothesis should be carried out and reviewed by competent institutional review boards.

The truth is, however, that there is *no* evidence from controlled studies which supports Dr. Crook's theory or method of treatment. His own work has not been subjected to peer review. Instead, it has been published in nonrefereed journals and in books published by a company called Professional Books, the phone number for which is the same as that for Dr. Crook's office.

In the single well-controlled study which explored the presumed relationship between sources of Candida in the body and the "candidiasis hypersensitivity syndrome," researchers concluded that 1) the syndrome itself cannot be verified; and 2) complaints supposedly associated with it do not respond to treatment with antifungal medication.[20] In fact, the researchers noted that Dr. Crook's treatment program contains so many components that there may be no way to submit this theory to controlled scientific investigation. How, for example, could an investigator control for factors which include a controlled diet, antifungal medication, possible food allergies, and exposure to antibiotics, tobacco smoke, diesel fumes, perfumes, environmental molds, and "poisons and pollutant of all kinds which contaminate the air, soil and water"? Since this is obviously an impossible task, proponents of this approach can always argue that critical factors were overlooked, making the results of the study meaningless.

*Dangers*

The mainstays of Dr. Crook's treatment program, a low-sugar diet and antifungal medication, do not appear to pose any danger to health. However, as we discussed in the section on orthomolecular approaches, there are documented hazards associated with excessive doses of vitamins and minerals.

*Conclusions*

Dr. Crook's theory and treatment approach appear to fall solidly in the category of wishful thinking. Unless and until this approach is subjected to rigorous scientific investigation, it should not be employed in the treatment of ADHD.

**ESSENTIAL FATTY ACIDS AND OIL OF EVENING PRIMROSE**

Fats are nutrients which provide the body with its most concentrated form of energy. Most of us are very well aware that diets too high in fat contribute not only to unwanted rolls and bulges but to many serious health problems, such as coronary heart disease and stroke.

Not all fats are bad, however. One group, known as *essential fatty acids (EFAs)*, are essential for maintaining health, as their name implies. EFAs are vital components of cell membranes and necessary building blocks of prostaglandins, hormone-like compounds which regulate many bodily functions. Since the body cannot make EFAs, they must be obtained from dietary sources. Certain vegetable oils are a good source of linolenic acid, the main Omega-6 fatty acid, while the oils of salmon and other cold-water fish are rich in alpha-linolenic acid, an Omega-3 fatty acid.

Deficiencies in EFAs have been suggested as the cause of numerous ailments, including premenstrual syndrome, arthritis, and atopic eczema. The notion that deficiencies in EFAs can cause ADHD has been promoted most strongly by the Hyperactive Children's Support Group, a British organization which also advocates use of the Feingold Diet and vitamin supplementation to treat ADHD.

What might cause a youngster to be deficient in EFAs? According to Dr. Leo Galland, coauthor *of Superimmunity for Kids*,[21] deficiencies in EFAs can result from a diet too high in sugar or refined flour, both of which increase the need for EFAs. A dietary surplus of hydrogenated vegetable oils, such as are found in margarine and crackers and other snack foods, can also interfere with EFA availability, as can a lack of certain enzymes, vitamins, or other substances necessary to process EFAs in the body. Finally, consistent with Dr. Crook's theory, chronic yeast infections are believed to interfere with fat metabolism and produce deficiencies in EFAs.

According to Dr. Galland, the child who is deficient in EFAs can be recognized by other symptoms, which include the following:

· Excessive thirst

· Dry, flaking skin; bumps on outer thighs, upper arms, cheeks

· Brittle, soft, or splitting fingernails

· Dry hair; dandruff

- Eczema, asthma, multiple allergies

Treatment for suspected EFA deficiency consists of a diet low in sugar, white flour, and hydrogenated fat, as well as dietary supplements of EFAs like flaxseed oil and cod liver oil. An EFA supplement which has attracted particular attention is oil of evening primrose, a rich source of gamma-linolenic acid derived from the seeds of the evening primrose plant. This poetic-sounding substance is manufactured under the trade name Efamol and is available in health food stores.

*The Evidence*

A deficiency of EFA intake has long been known to produce severe skin disorders, and several studies have reported promising results using EFA supplements such as Efamol in the treatment of atopic eczema and other skin conditions. This approach is also under study as an adjunctive treatment in other medical conditions, including rheumatoid arthritis.

Is there reason to believe that deficiencies in EFAs might also play a role in ADHD? This hypothesis seems rather far-fetched in light of what we know about ADHD, although one study has reported lower serum levels of EFAs in a group of children with ADHD in comparison with a control group.[22]

In 1981, a study conducted in England under the auspices of the Hyperactive Children's Support Group reported dramatic improvement in several ADHD children treated with oil of evening primrose.[23] As the authors noted, however, their studies were not controlled in any way, so we must consider the results only as anecdotal evidence.

Subsequently, two well-controlled studies using a double-blind design were conducted in the United States.[24, 25] In both studies, the results did not support Efamol as an effective treatment for ADHD.

*Conclusions*

Although we know of no dangers associated with dietary supplementation of EFAs, Efamol is expensive. Since there is no evidence suggesting that it is helpful to children with ADHD, the cost does not seem justified and we cannot recommend it as a treatment for ADHD.

**AMINO ACIDS**

When we eat meat, fish, eggs, and other high-protein foods, our digestive system first breaks the proteins in these foods into smaller particles called "peptides" and, ultimately, into even smaller units called "amino acids." These amino acids are then used by the body to create hormones, enzymes, and substances which promote the healing of wounds and build and maintain the immune system.

More important, for our purposes, amino acids are components of neurotransmitters, the chemical messengers in the brain. The amino acid phenylalanine, for example, is necessary in the synthesis of dopamine and norepinephrine, two important neurotransmitters. Tryptophan is essential in the manufacture of serotonin, another important neurotransmitter.

There are twenty amino acids which are essential for the growth and maintenance of the body. Twelve of them can be manufactured by the body, but the other eight, called "essential," must be supplied from dietary sources.

Since foods eventually become neurotransmitters, some investigators have reasoned that brain function depends heavily on diets which contain the right amounts of amino acids. Accordingly, it has been suggested that phenylalanine, tyrosine, and tryptophan might be used as alternative treatments for ADHD.

*The Evidence*

Since it is well established that amino acids are important constituents of neurotransmitters and since neurotransmitter malfunctions have clearly been implicated in ADHD, this theory certainly has logical appeal. It also gains some credence, in a roundabout way, from the fact that perturbations in the body's ability to process amino acids are known to have very serious consequences for brain function. Phenylketonuria (PKU), for example, a condition which results in brain damage and mental retardation, occurs when the body cannot break down phenylalanine. Treatment of PKU consists of, among other things, a diet low in phenylalanine.

What about the evidence for amino acid supplementation as a treatment for ADHD? While the theory seems to make good sense—like so many other theories we have discussed—the evidence does not support it. To date, at least three studies of amino acid supplementation have been published, with disappointing results. In two of these investigations, the use of phenylalanine was explored; and in one, the effects of tryptophan and tyrosine were evaluated.[26, 27, 28] Taken together, the findings indicate that amino acid supplementation is *not* helpful in the treatment of ADHD.

*Conclusions*

Although the theory concerning amino acid supplementation for treating children with ADHD is compelling, the evidence is not. This treatment should not be employed with youngsters who have ADHD.

**OTHER MEDICATIONS**

*Piracetam*

Piracetam (pyrrolidine acetamide) is a relatively new drug which is structurally related to gamma-aminobutyric acid (GABA), a neurotransmitter in the central nervous system. It is neither a stimulant nor a sedative, and it appears to be quite safe, with few, if any, side effects. In Europe, it is marketed under the names Nootrop and Nootropil. In the United States, it is considered an experimental drug and therefore is not commercially available.

*The Evidence*

Early investigations of its effects on verbal learning in humans were conducted on college-student volunteers. When results were promising, piracetam was then tested on reading-disabled children. These studies used sound scientific methods of investigation, and the majority of them showed that piracetam produced some improvement in reading skills.

The most impressive of these studies was a multisite endeavor which involved researchers at centers affiliated with five major universities in the United States. In this well-controlled study, 225 dyslexic children were given piracetam or a placebo for a thirty-six-week period. Results showed consistent improvements in reading speed, accuracy, and comprehension.[29]

*Conclusions*

Piracetam is not a miracle drug. Even though some reading-disabled children seem to benefit from it, they still do not become "normal" readers. There is also at least one well-controlled study in which no beneficial effects of piracetam were found.[30] Nevertheless, this is a very promising approach, one which certainly merits continued study.

## Chapter 7

### Dietary Interventions

As treatments for childhood learning and behavior problems, few approaches are more controversial than those which involve special diets. The battle lines have been drawn and emotions run high on both sides of the diet debate. Proponents of dietary modification claim that 50 percent of children with learning or attention problems can be cured by their methods, with another 25 percent showing considerable improvement. Critics of this approach point to the lack of convincing scientific data. In turn, proponents argue that thousands of children have been helped by their methods and ask "Why should we have to prove what so many parents already know?"

We don't know how many children are currently on some type of controlled diet for their learning or behavior problems, but we do know that the subject of dietary intervention has consistently attracted a great deal of public interest over the years. This interest is apparent each time an article is published in the popular press or a spokesperson for the dietary approach appears on a television talk show. Physician Doris Rapp, for example, has been a frequent guest on "Donahue." In fact, she actually dedicated her recent book, *Is This Your Child? Discovering and Treating Unrecognized Allergies*,[1] to Phil Donahue "with thanks and appreciation to Phil and his staff for the opportunity to share so much information, which changed the lives of so many children and their families. BLESS YOU FOR HELPING SO MANY!"

Even respected scientists like Dr. Keith Conners, developer of the widely used Conners Scales, have fueled the controversy. In his book *Feeding the Brain*,[2] he concludes that "to some extent ... parents and teachers must become experimenters themselves because they cannot wait for resolution of all conflicting evidence."

**ARE YOU WHAT YOU EAT?**

The belief that the food we eat affects how we think, feel, and behave is instilled early in our lives. Remember Mom insisting that you eat a healthful diet and her exhortation to "think about the starving children in China"?

But we are not discussing malnutrition when we talk about dietary intervention for learning and behavior problems. Malnutrition at any age produces documented effects on learning and behavior, and if malnutrition occurs during the first year of life, the effects on intellectual development and behavior can be permanent. Most children in the developed world do not suffer from malnutrition, however, nor do the majority of those with learning and attention problems have histories of severe malnutrition.

Since most American children do not suffer from malnutrition, why do we continue to suspect that diet plays such a major role in learning disabilities and behavior problems? As we discussed in Chapter 6, it has long been known that many of the chemical substances used by the brain are supplied by dietary sources. Therefore, some have reasoned, manipulation of diet *might* have an effect on these brain chemicals. In turn, the amount of these chemicals available to the brain *might* affect behavior and learning. Tryptophan, for example, which is present in foods like turkey and milk, is one of the building blocks used by the brain to produce the neurotransmitter serotonin, known to affect mood, attention, and learning. If we eat lots of foods known to be high in serotonin, *might* we thereby improve our mood and increase our capacity to learn?

And just as it seems reasonable to assume that increasing the availability of certain chemicals might enhance brain functioning, isn't is also possible that there are substances which have detrimental effects on the brain? Certainly, as we have become more knowledgeable about the environmental hazards around us, we have become increasingly wary of pollutants, chemicals, and food additives. How do we know, for example, that food additives are really safe?

Since over four thousand chemicals are used in food processing, some of them *might* adversely affect the brain. And what about refined sugar? If problems regulating blood sugar can produce the devastating effects seen in diabetes, isn't it possible that diets high in refined sugar *might* interfere with the complex brain activity associated with learning and behavior?

All of this sounds reasonable, but from a scientific perspective, there are just too many "mights" involved. This has not, however, deterred proponents of dietary intervention from touting speculations as fact, nor has it led them to moderate their claim that many serious problems will respond to dietary treatment. In the following sections, we will review the most popular of these approaches and examine the evidence concerning their effectiveness.

**ADDITIVE-FREE DIETS**

Interest in dietary manipulation to treat children's learning and behavior problems can be traced largely to the influence of the late Dr. Ben Feingold, a pediatrician and allergist who practiced in California. Over twenty years ago, Dr. Feingold observed that children who were sensitive to aspirin often had similar reactions to food colorings and to salicylates, the acidic substances that give many fruits their tangy flavor. Over time, he expanded his list of offending substances to include artificial flavorings and preservatives.

Dr. Feingold never explained exactly how these substances work in the brain to affect learning and behavior. Nevertheless, he speculated that reactions to these substances were responsible for about half the cases of ADHD in this country and proposed an additive-free diet to treat ADHD. He claimed that when ADHD children were placed on his controlled diet, approximately half showed such "dramatic" improvement that they were able to discontinue stimulants and other medications within ten days. He also claimed that significant improvements in academic performance could be observed within a single quarter at school.

With the appearance of his book *Why Your Child Is Hyperactive*,[3] Feingold's theory and his diet were greeted with enthusiasm by the public. Feingold Associations, comprised mainly of parents, were formed in almost every state to disseminate information about the diet and to provide support for parents who chose to use Feingold's approach with their children.

*The Evidence*

The list of foods and other substances which contain additives, dyes, or salicylates is an impressive one indeed. But when we consider the evidence for an additive-free diet as a treatment for children's learning and behavior problems, we End that it is very much less than impressive.

Unfortunately, Dr. Feingold did not provide evidence from scientific studies to support his theories or his claims. Instead, he offered only a great deal of anecdotal evidence from his own clinical experience, as well as testimonials from parents who had tried his approach and found it helpful for their children.

In 1982, in response to controversy surrounding Dr. Feingold's claims, the National Institutes of Health held a three-day conference on the relationship between additive-free diets and ADHD.[4] At this conference, a panel of experts concluded that there *might* be a very small group of hyperactive children who respond to additive-free diets. However, they cautioned that even in this group, the results of additive-free diets are still much less impressive than claimed by proponents of this approach.

A few years later, physician and researcher Dr. Esther Wender reviewed the studies which had been done to that point. She found that most of the studies which claimed to identify a diet-behavior relationship were quite seriously flawed, and she concluded that "these studies generally refute a causal association between food additives and behavioral disturbance in children."[5]

What about the few studies in which a relationship between an additive-free diet and behavior has been found? In some research studies, children showed no improvement in behavior on the Feingold Diet when it was presented *before* the control (sham) diet. Only when the Feingold Diet was presented *after* the control diet did parents and teachers report improved behavior on the Feingold Diet. Apparently, the difference between the two diets became obvious to the participants, so we cannot be sure whether perceived improvement stemmed from the diet or from the placebo effect.

Somewhat more convincing evidence has come from so-called "challenge" studies in which children on an additive-free diet are given "challenge" doses of additives and subsequent changes in behavior are assessed. Two such studies have lent some support to the belief that food dyes can have an adverse effect on the behavior of some children.[6, 7] In these double-blind studies, a total of seventy-seven ADHD children were challenged with artificial food coloring. Three children consistently showed worsening of symptoms in response to food colorings. Of these three children, one was below the age of three and two suffered from asthma and other allergies.

*Conclusions*

Taken together, the results of these studies suggest that as the NIH panel concluded, there may be a small group of children who respond negatively to artificial food coloring as if it were a drug or a toxic substance. As Dr. Keith Conners has observed, if one of these children is your child, you won't care very much about statistics. Nevertheless, parents need to know that the likelihood that an ADHD child's problems can be corrected by removing additives from his diet is quite small indeed.

**ALLERGEN-FREE DIETS**

Today, although enthusiasm for the Feingold Diet has waned considerably in our society, the presumed connection between diet and behavior is by no means dead. Now, however, proponents of this theory cite specific allergies—especially food allergies—as the most common cause of learning and behavior problems in children.[*]

Currently, Dr. Doris Rapp is probably the best-known advocate of dietary modification as a means of treating learning and behavior problems. Dr. Rapp is a pediatrician and an allergist who practices in Buffalo, New York. She has written several books on the relationship between allergies and learning/behavior problems and, as mentioned, has appeared repeatedly on television talk shows.

According to Dr. Rapp, the number of children and adults who suffer from allergies or sensitivities to foods and environmental substances may exceed three quarters of the population of the United States. Potentially offending substances, she claims, are found not only in the foods we eat but in the water we drink, the medicines and cosmetics we use, the clothes we wear, the houses we live in—even (especially!) the air we breathe.

Dr. Rapp claims that unrecognized allergies to foods and environmental substances are the cause of a host of human ailments. Her list goes far beyond such well-known allergy-related symptoms as hives, eczema, and respiratory problems. Although she issues the disclaimer "No, everything is not an allergy," she goes on to cite symptoms as diverse as joint stiffness, fatigue, headaches, stomach ailments, seizures, sleep problems, fecal soiling, alcoholism, and obesity. She implicates unrecognized allergies as a cause not only of learning and behavior problems such as ADHD but of Tourette's syndrome, depression, and even suicide. Concerning her claim that allergies are significantly more common among adopted children, she goes so far as to speculate that many of these infants may have "cried so much because of an undetected milk allergy that the mother was overwhelmed and placed the infant for adoption."[8]

Under child behaviors which might signal an allergic reaction, she lists an impressive array which includes temper tantrums, whining, screaming, clinging, hyperactivity, aggression, repetition of the same phrases, nonstop senseless talk, reluctance to smile, excessive fatigue, depression, refusal to stay dressed, refusal to be touched, and desire to crouch in dark corners or hide under furniture.

How does Dr. Rapp propose to treat the many problems which she claims are caused by unrecognized allergies? She recommends that parents who suspect an allergy- or sensitivity-related problem begin by observing their child closely to identify relationships between various substances which the child has eaten or with which he has come into contact ("What did he drink, eat, smell or touch?") and the onset of symptoms.

This observation period may be followed by allergy testing, using the method known as "provocation/neutralization" (P/N). In P/N testing, small amounts of potentially allergenic items are injected into the upper layers of the child's skin (provocation). If there is a skin reaction or if the child's symptoms are reproduced, the test is considered positive. The "provoked" symptoms are then stopped by administering a weaker solution of the same test item (neutralization).

If chemical sensitivities appear to be the source of the problem, blood or urine tests may be in order, as well as specific tests to measure levels of some chemicals in the immediate environment. If food allergies are suspected, Dr. Rapp suggests an elimination diet. As we explained in an earlier section, an elimination diet involves removing the suspected foods for a period of time and observing behavior changes. Offending foods are then reintroduced and the child is observed to see whether behavior worsens in response.

Depending on the individual patient, Dr. Rapp may recommend a course of allergy extract therapy. In traditional allergy treatment programs, allergy extracts are injected under the skin in progressively stronger concentrations at regular intervals over a period of many months. Dr. Rapp's preferred method, however, is to use minute amounts of allergy extract, placed under the patient's tongue ("sublingual"). Sometimes this method is combined with the subcutaneous (under-the-skin) method.

Other elements in a treatment program may include allergy-proofing the environment, avoiding exposure to offending chemicals, and eliminating offending chemicals already stored in the body through a variety of detoxification procedures.

Concerning learning disabilities, Dr. Rapp cites many examples of youngsters with school problems who showed dramatic improvement when treated with her methods. Blaming unrecognized allergies and sensitivities for many cases of ADHD, she cites her own 1978 study in which 65 percent of a group of hyperactive youngsters on Ritalin were helped by her methods "without the use of any pills or drugs."[9]

*The Evidence*

There is no doubt that Dr. Rapp's approach to treating children with ADHD and learning disabilities has tremendous popular appeal. The solutions she proposes appear to be simple to implement and quick to produce dramatic results. The methods she employs combine what sounds like the latest in high-tech medicine—so new, in fact, that few professionals are as yet familiar with them—and a "natural" (nondrug) approach to treatment. This is a combination which seems to combine the best of both worlds. But does it work? Does Dr. Rapp's approach really help children with learning and behavior problems? Before we examine the evidence, let's ask a few basic questions about her theories and methods.

**Current Concepts in ADHD.** Turning first to the area of ADHD, we find that Dr. Rapp's assertions concerning ADHD and Ritalin are not consistent with current thinking in the field. She states, for example, that "ecologists have found such a definite overlap between ADHD and ATFS [Allergic Tension Fatigue Syndrome] that they often appear to be in the same mixed bag."[10] She does not, however, provide any data to substantiate this claim. Implying that parents who give their ADHD children Ritalin do so selfishly, because it is "easy," she cautions that Ritalin is addictive and warns that if it is stopped abruptly or even gradually decreased and stopped, it can cause fatigue, disturbed sleep, depression, Tourette's syndrome, psychosis, or suicide.[11] Finally, she inaccurately depicts the Citizens Commission on Human Rights as a group of crusaders on an educational mission without a closer examination of their motives.

**Current Theories in Allergy Medicine.** Similarly, Dr. Rapp's theories and methods do not accord with what is generally accepted practice in allergy medicine. Much of what she proposes is very much outside the mainstream of current thinking, including her contentions that:

· Allergies affect global rather than specific areas of the body.

· Allergies do not have to be due to established and acceptable causes.

· Allergies do not need to be scientifically confirmed in order to be recognized.

Further, as she herself points out, "Most allergists do not believe in P/N testing."[12] In this assertion, she is correct: over a decade ago the American Academy of Allergy and Immunology issued a position statement rejecting the provocation/neutralization method, whether subcutaneous or sublingual, as a method for either diagnosing or treating allergies.[13] To date, the American Academy of Allergy and Immunology has not seen fit to alter its stance.

How does Dr. Rapp explain the fact that her approach has failed to gain acceptance within her own profession? Citing "the powerful pharmaceutical, food, and/or chemical industries," she states that "the bottom line, unfortunately, appears possibly to be vested interests."[14] In other words, Dr. Rapp believes that a conspiracy exists to prevent physicians from learning about, and using, a technique which could help many of their patients.

All of these objections might be less worrisome if there were evidence from well-controlled studies which supported Dr. Rapp's claims. But this is not the case. Instead of such evidence, Dr. Rapp provides only anecdotes and case studies. At this time, there are no well-controlled studies in which her approach has been evaluated and shown to be helpful to youngsters with learning and behavior problems.

**Other Lines of Evidence.** But let's be careful not to throw out the proverbial baby with the bath water! While Dr. Rapp's approach has not been proven, it would be premature to conclude that there is no evidence linking food allergies to children's problems. In fact, recent research conducted in England and Canada suggests that food allergies and sensitivities *may* contribute to behavior problems and physical symptoms, *at least in a select group of children.*

In England, Dr. Joseph Egger and his colleagues placed a group of seventy-six children on an oligoandgenic diet; that is, a diet limited to only a few foods.[15] Improvement was reported in sixty-two children during this "open" (nonblind) phase. These children were then challenged with regular foods, including additives, to identify problem substances for each child. A group for whom problem substances were identified were then exposed, in double-blind fashion, to the offending substances and to a placebo. Although no differences were found in psychological test scores, parents and other observers reported that behavior problems and other symptoms were significantly worse when the children received the offending substances than when they received a placebo. Several children also showed considerable improvement in a variety of other troublesome symptoms, including headaches and seizures.

More recently, Dr. Bonnie Kaplan's group at the University of Calgary also found evidence for a diet-behavior link in a group of hyperactive preschoolers with known allergies.[16] Dr. Kaplan placed these children on a diet free of additives, chocolate, MSG, caffeine, and other substances to which individual children in the study were thought to be sensitive (for example, dairy products). As a result of this double-blind study, ten of the twenty-four youngsters improved by 25 percent or more in terms of behavior ratings. There were also improvements in physical symptoms, including headaches and rhinitis, as well as in sleep problems.

The results of these studies are certainly fascinating, but before we all rush to put our children on exotic diets, a few words of caution are in order. It is vitally important to stress that neither Dr. Egger nor Dr. Kaplan studied youngsters with "garden-variety" ADHD. From a group of 196 preschoolers referred for hyperactivity, Dr. Kaplan selected only 24, all with allergic symptoms and sleep problems in addition to ADHD. Dr. Egger's group included many youngsters with developmental delays, mental retardation, seizures, recurrent headaches and stomachaches, skin rashes, mouth ulcers, and other symptoms not typical of children with ADHD. Thus, in neither study could the children be considered representative of ADHD children in general.

*Conclusions*

The evidence to date suggests that there is a small group of children who have multiple physical and behavioral difficulties in addition to symptoms of ADHD who may benefit from dietary intervention. The children most likely to respond are those who are *quite young* and who *suffer from myriad problems besides ADHD*, including allergies, sleep disorders, and a variety of neurological problems. However, we *cannot* conclude that most—or even many—children with ADHD will respond favorably to dietary intervention.

It is also important to stress that the diets employed by Drs. Egger and Kaplan are not without dangers and drawbacks. As Dr. Egger cautioned, this method should be considered only for severely affected children because:

- There are no specific diagnostic tests.

- It is difficult to apply, as well as expensive and disruptive to the social life of children and families.

- Trained staff must monitor the diet, which, unsupervised, is potentially dangerous.

- Some parents may use the diet in a punitive fashion.

Concerning Dr. Rapp's specific approach, there is no evidence from well-controlled scientific studies which supports its effectiveness as a treatment for children with learning and behavior problems. Further, we believe that there are some potential dangers associated with this approach to treating ADHD and learning-disabled children. As clinical psychologists, we are particularly concerned about the list of "symptoms" which Dr. Rapp believes are allergy-related. Our combined forty-five years' experience in working with children suggests that some of these symptoms actually signal the presence of serious emotional disturbance, while others suggest possible psychological consequences of physical or sexual abuse.

Cost factors in terms of both time and money are also a cause for concern. Dr. Rapp states that P/N testing can be very time-consuming; that, in fact, three to six full days of constant testing and supervision may be required in complicated cases. Since, as she acknowledges, these procedures are often not covered by insurance, the cost can represent a significant financial drain on families of modest means. If families must then forgo exploring other means of helping their ADHD or learning-disabled children, this represents a real disservice to these youngsters. Therefore, we cannot recommend Dr. Rapp's approach to parents of children with ADHD and learning disabilities.

**SUGAR-FREE DIETS**

Sugar, in all its myriad forms, might be aptly described as "the stuff we love to hate." At the same time that we consume about 130 pounds per person per year, we blame refined sugar for everything from hyperactivity to homicidal impulses: remember the "Twinkies defense" put forth by Dan White, who claimed that he killed the mayor and the supervisor of San Francisco while under the influence of the sugar contained in several Twinkies?

In a society in which two major holidays (Halloween and Easter) are specifically associated with receiving and consuming large amounts of candy, there is no doubt that American children do indeed ingest quite a bit of refined sugar. And there is probably not a parent in America who wouldn't swear to the fact that his children are particularly wild on Halloween. Professionals, too, share this opinion: when pediatricians and family practitioners were surveyed a few years ago, almost half of the respondents stated that they sometimes recommended a sugar-restricted diet for their hyperactive patients.[17]

Is sugar really a "toxin," as some have called it? Certainly, there are many who think that this is the case. Sugar, we are told, causes worsening of hyperactivity and distractibility in ADHD children and can adversely affect behavior in non-ADHD children as well. There are even those who have postulated a link between sugar and violent antisocial behavior: in studies of prisoners incarcerated for violent crimes, some researchers have claimed reductions in hostility and aggressive behavior when prisoners have been placed on sugar-restricted diets.

There is disagreement, however, concerning the exact manner in which sugar might act on the brain to produce abnormalities in behavior. Dr. Doris Rapp, for example, believes that some children suffer allergic responses to sugar, while Dr. William Crook (see Chapter 6) thinks that it exerts harmful effects by stimulating excessive yeast growth within the body. Some researchers have speculated that sugar influences the levels of certain neurotransmitters, such as serotonin, in the central nervous system, while others have suggested that sugar interferes with the ability of fatty acids to synthesize necessary substances within the brain. Still others—especially those who see a connection between sugar and violent crime—lay the blame on hypoglycemia, a condition in which glucose levels in the blood are abnormally low.

*The Evidence*

How much do we really know about the effects of sugar on human behavior? Is there a relationship between sugar intake and hyperactive, aggressive behavior? If there is, what can we conclude about the nature of this relationship?

Although there is a large body of literature devoted to this subject, many of the reports reflect only the speculations of the authors or their clinical observations, unsubstantiated by any kind of scientific data. In more rigorous studies, scientists have used two methods to examine the relationship between sugar and behavior. Using the *correlational method*, some have tried to identify a connection ("co-relation") between a child's behavior patterns and the average amount of sugar in his diet. In *intervention studies*, researchers have actively manipulated the amount of dietary sugar and then observed subsequent effects on behavior.

In a widely cited correlational study done in 1980,[18] researchers obtained seven-day diet records on a group of ADHD children and a group of normal children. In analyzing the diet records and comparing behavior observed in the laboratory, they found that higher levels of sugar consumption were associated with higher levels of restlessness in both groups of children. In the ADHD group, high sugar consumption was also associated with higher levels of aggressive behavior.

This study was hailed as "proof" that sugar adversely affects behavior. However, other scientists found fault with some of the methods used, and when the study was repeated by another group using more precise methods of measuring dietary sugar, the connections between sugar and behavior were *not* found.[19]

Of course, correlational studies—whatever the results—cannot be used to determine cause-and-effect relationships. If hyperactive children really do consume more sugar than other children, does this mean that sugar causes hyperactive behavior? Or does it simply mean that hyperactive children need higher levels of sugar because they bounce around so much?

In an attempt to answer these questions, other scientists have actively manipulated the amount of dietary sugar and then observed subsequent effects on behavior. Some researchers have observed children's behavior in the laboratory setting,[20, 21] while others have tackled the more arduous task of studying behavior in the natural environment of home, classroom, and playground.[22] Some of these studies have been quite ambitious in scope: psychologists Richard Milich and William Pelham, for example, examined the effects of sugar on twenty-five different aspects of child behavior, including academic productivity and accuracy, social behavior, on-task behavior, rule violations, and body movements.[23]

*Conclusions*

Taken together, the results of these studies can be summarized as follows:

- There is no convincing evidence that sugar has marked adverse effects on the behavior of elementary-school-age children, including children with ADHD. A few well-designed studies have found some effects of sugar on behavior, but these are very small and only a small percentage of children seems to be vulnerable. Even Dr. Keith Conners, who has identified such effects in his own research, flatly states, "None of the findings in sugar studies justify eliminating sugar from the diet of children."[24]

- If adverse behavioral effects of sugar do exist, they may be more evident in a some very young (pre-school-age) children. Even here, however, the effects reported have been small in magnitude.

Based on these conclusions, we do not recommend sugar-restricted diets as an approach to treating children with ADHD. In the daily life of the ADHD child, already fraught with so many problems, it simply does not make sense to use an unproven approach that may provide nothing more than additional opportunities for parent-child conflict.

This said, two caveats are in order. First, we do not mean to imply that general nutrition is unimportant. Like all children, children with learning and attention problems need healthful, well-balanced diets. Many researchers, including Dr. Conners, have given us reason to believe that a good breakfast is particularly important and that, to be most helpful, breakfast should be high in protein. While many ADHD children are picky eaters, even they can be encouraged to eat a good breakfast if it is packaged in the form of a sandwich (peanut butter, tuna fish, grilled cheese, turkey are all good sources of protein) or that all-time childhood favorite, pizza.

Second, we should note that some rare children really do seem to have abnormal cravings for sugar and other carbohydrates. These children will go to virtually any lengths, including theft, to obtain carbohydrates. They frequently consume large amounts of sweets at a single sitting and attempt to hide the evidence of consumption (wrappers, boxes, and so on). They may also hoard caches of cookies, candy, and other high-carbohydrate foods.

In our clinical experience, these children are apt to be suffering from mood disorders (depression) rather than ADHD alone. In fact, Dr. Norman Rosenthal and his colleagues at the National Institute of Mental Health have actually identified a particular type of recurrent depression which is associated with very pronounced carbohydrate cravings and subsequent weight gain.[25] If you are convinced that your child has abnormal cravings for carbohydrates, we suggest that you look into possible underlying causes before attempting to treat the symptoms by restricting the child's access to sugar.

* Unlike the condition known as "sensitivity," in which the body responds to a substance as if it were poisonous, an "allergy" refers to a condition in which the body responds to certain substances by producing specific antibodies. These antibodies are responsible for the release of histamines, which, in turn, produce allergic symptoms.

## Chapter 8

### Training Approaches to Treatment

Approaches which use training methods to help children overcome learning and attention problems are particularly likely to find favor in our culture. We are, after all, a people who believe fervently in self-improvement. We believe in willpower and self-control, and we venerate people who have overcome adversity to bring themselves up by their proverbial bootstraps. So, when we are offered a treatment approach which promises to train our children in better ways of behaving and learning, it isn't at all surprising that we would respond with optimism and enthusiasm.

What are these training approaches? What do we know about them? Most important, can they really help our children?

**EEG BIOFEEDBACK:
TRAINING THE BRAIN**

The term "biofeedback" refers to a technique in which a person is taught to use information about a normally involuntary body function, such as heart rate or blood pressure, to gain voluntary control over that function. Biofeedback procedures involve measuring activity in a specific organ or system of the body and transforming this information into a signal like a light or a tone. Using this signal as "feedback," the patient is then trained to alter the level of activity in the desired direction. If, for example, we wanted to induce relaxation by decreasing muscle tension in certain areas of the body, electromyographic (EMG) feedback from these muscle groups would be given in the form of a signal informing the patient when levels of activity were in the target range. With practice, the patient learns to produce consistent low levels of activity in the selected muscle groups and, in so doing, achieves deep levels of relaxation.[*]

Recently, the notion that ADHD children can be helped by using electroencephalography (EEG) biofeedback techniques to correct faulty patterns of brain electrical activity has received a great deal of attention in the popular press. Articles in *Woman's Day*[1] and *Reader's Digest*[2] have touted EEG biofeedback as a scientific breakthrough and a sure cure for learning and attention problems. Readers are led to believe that within a few short years, these troublesome childhood disorders will be virtually eliminated through the use of these techniques.

The idea of using EEG biofeedback with ADHD children is not new. Over fifteen years ago, Dr. Joel Lubar, a psychologist on the faculty at the University of Tennessee, published a case study in which one "hyperkinetic" (ADHD) child was successfully treated with this method.[3] Since that time, additional articles have appeared in professional journals, all reporting dramatic success in treating the multiple problems of children with ADHD.

Exactly what is EEG biofeedback and how is it supposed to work? Electroencephalography is a technique in which wires attached to the skull are used to detect and record "brain waves," patterns of electrical activity produced by large numbers of brain cells. Certain of these patterns are associated with seizure disorders (epilepsy) and other pathological conditions. Other patterns are associated with certain kinds of mental activity. Alpha waves, for example, occur when a person is relaxed and calm, while beta waves are associated with an alert state of concentration and mental effort. Delta waves occur in sleep, and theta waves are the slow waves which are the predominant pattern in very young children.

For many years, scientists have debated whether differences exist in the brain-wave patterns of children with and without ADHD. Early research efforts involved simply "eyeballing" the paper tracings of brain activity, scanning for clear-cut abnormalities. These efforts were generally disappointing, with some investigators claiming to spot differences which others failed to find.[4]

More recently, scientists have availed themselves of improved technology to study this issue. Using up-to-the- minute computer analysis techniques, researchers have indeed found differences in patterns of brain-wave activity between ADHD youngsters and other children. Specifically, they have found that in comparison with their age-mates, children with ADHD produce abnormally high levels of theta activity and abnormally low levels of beta waves, especially in the frontal regions of the brain—the same regions in which brain-imaging techniques have revealed lower levels of arousal.[5, 6]

This, then, is the idea behind EEG biofeedback: using biofeedback techniques, ADHD children are trained to increase brain waves presumed to be associated with focused attention (beta waves) and to decrease brain waves claimed to be associated with daydreaming (theta waves). This is done by gluing a number of electrodes to the child's scalp to record brain electrical activity. This information is fed into a computer, which transforms it into a signal. The child then uses this signal as feedback and earns rewards for producing increased amounts of the desired brainwave activity. The child is also encouraged to sit very still during training sessions, since movement interferes with the ability of the equipment to detect brain waves. Often, explicit instructions for relaxation are given, and because these and other components are included in the overall program, Dr. Lubar has recently renamed his approach "neurotherapy."

About forty to eighty treatment sessions are usually required, with each session lasting forty minutes or so. Since sessions are typically provided two to three times per week, treatment can extend over three to ten months or even longer. Dr. Lubar's program also includes regular academic tutoring sessions and family consultation.

After all of this, what kind of results should we expect? The claims made by proponents of this approach are certainly impressive. We are told that intelligence test scores can increase by as many as 33 points; that grade point averages typically increase by 1.5 levels; that the average increase in grade level is 2.5 years; and that, after training, 60 percent of ADHD children no longer require medication.[7] Some who practice this approach have also reported significant improvements in handwriting and manual dexterity and even changes in a child's requirements for prescriptive lenses.[8] Finally, it is claimed that results obtained with EEG biofeedback are permanent, a claim which is most impressive in light of the fact that *no* treatment currently available for ADHD has been shown to produce permanent benefit when the treatment is discontinued.

*The Evidence*

It is no wonder that this approach has attracted so much attention recently. This is heady stuff indeed! Why, then, haven't clinicians and scientists scrambled to provide this form of therapy for ADHD children? After all, as supporters of neurotherapy point out, their theory is quite consistent with what is known about low levels of arousal in frontal brain areas in individuals with ADHD. And, as we noted, there is documentation that the brain-wave patterns of ADHD children do differ from those of other children.

But before we go any further, let's examine this premise a little more closely. The approach seems logical: change the abnormal patterns of brain-wave activity and thereby change the condition itself. Once again, however, it is quite possible that the relationship between cause and effect has been confused; that is, the abnormal patterns of brain electrical activity in ADHD children might be a *byproduct* of the condition rather than a *cause* of it.

An analogy might help to clarify things at this point. If we were to observe a group of people suffering from depression, we would certainly see that they smiled far less frequently than people who are not depressed. Suppose we then trained our depressed patients to increase their rate of smiling by giving them a dollar every time they smiled. If we wanted to go high-tech, we could even use EMG biofeedback, targeting the facial musculature and providing feedback and rewards for increases in activity in those muscles which control smiling. While it is a pretty sure bet that we could increase smiling using these techniques, it's not very likely that we would have cured, or even improved, the underlying depression in these patients.

Returning to the issue of EEG biofeedback, several studies have demonstrated that children trained with this technique quickly learn to alter their brain-wave patterns in the desired direction. Can we be sure, however, that this is the cause for the reported improvements in learning and behavior? Even some professionals who advocate this approach and who use it themselves think otherwise. Dr. Dennis Kade, for example, a psychologist who studied with Dr. Lubar and who himself uses EEG biofeedback with ADHD children, notes that there are several other components which are included in the package known as "neurotherapy."[9]

How do we know that it is not these other components of the treatment package which actually produce the highly touted results? The answer is, we *don't* know that this is the case, and until we know otherwise, it is difficult to justify the use of a component as expensive as EEG biofeedback.

We also can't rule out our old nemesis, the placebo effect. Of all the treatments we have discussed so far, few are more likely to maximize this effect. The treatment itself is more than a bit impressive to a parent: there is your child, seated in a chair in a laboratory setting, his head connected to a spiderweb of wires—maybe even swathed in bandages to hold all the wiring in place—with lab-coated attendants turning dials and taking notes.

Even if you are not impressed by all the scientific trappings, you are sure to be impressed by the bill, since the cost of the entire course of training ranges between $3,000 and $6,000. Why should this figure into the equation by which you evaluate the outcome? Many years ago, social scientists observed that the more effort and expense a person puts into an endeavor, the greater the value he will assign to its outcome. This effect, known as "cognitive dissonance," would certainly seem to have some significance for the way in which parents who invest in biofeedback are predisposed to evaluate the results.

When we turn to scientific studies, what do we find? Despite the claims of Dr. Lubar and others that hundreds—even thousands—of ADHD children have been treated successfully with neurotherapy, the evidence supporting these claims is not very substantial. Published reports have included only a small number of children, and it is not clear to what extent these children could be considered ADHD or learning-disabled.

In terms of studies using double-blind controls, the evidence is not only scant but actually nonexistent. Proponents of this approach argue that it is not feasible to conduct such studies, since the professional who provides the treatment must remain closely involved to adjust the feedback throughout the training. Yet, in other studies of the application of biofeedback, "false feedback" has served as an appropriate placebo-control condition, so this objection seems somewhat questionable.

*Conclusions*

Biofeedback technology is not new. When it first appeared in the 1960s, it was hailed as a promising treatment for a host of human illnesses and ailments. Behavioral scientists and physicians were understandably excited about the idea that people could gain control over bodily processes and, by doing so, could literally learn to be healthy instead of sick.

Twenty-five years later, however, we find that biofeedback has not lived up to its early promise. Today, it serves as an ancillary treatment, usually used only in support of other treatments. As a treatment for chronic pain, it provides documented benefits, but the relief it offers is often no greater than that provided by simple relaxation methods. For disorders in which drugs are helpful, the drugs usually yield better results.

We think that the application of EEG biofeedback methods to the treatment of ADHD merits continued research efforts. Perhaps in the future a protocol will be developed which will prove to be effective with ADHD children. Until that time, however, it is a very expensive approach, the effectiveness of which has not yet been demonstrated. Until that time, too, we believe that advertising EEG biofeedback treatment as a "proven, non-pharmacological treatment for attention deficit disorder [10] is quite misleading. We caution parents, as consumers, to be appropriately skeptical about these claims.

**COGNITIVE THERAPY:**
**TRAINING THE MIND**

If we are to believe comedians and cartoonists, people who talk to themselves are either senile or suffering from serious mental illness. Psychologists, however, see it differently. Over a century ago, pioneering psychologist William James suggested that talking to oneself (he called this "self-directed speech") could be used to help people alter and control their own behavior. Since then, psychologists have developed a number of "cognitive" techniques to change people's behavior by teaching them to think differently.

Many of the cognitive strategies in widespread use today are based upon the work of the late Russian psychologists A. R. Luria[11] and L. Vygotsky.[12] Drs. Luria and Vygotsky studied the development of self-control in children and observed that it takes place in three stages. In the earliest stage, the toddler's behavior is controlled by external sources; that is, parents and others give the child explicit instructions, such as "No, no, don't touch," "That's hot," "Don't touch."

In the second stage, the child begins to control his own behavior by reminding himself of these instructions, actually reciting them aloud. Thus, the two-year-old approaching a hot stove is heard to say to himself "No, no, hot" as he tentatively extends and then withdraws his hand. In the third and final stage, the child appears to have internalized these instructions; that is, he no longer needs to hear a parental voice or even the sound of his own voice in order to recall the rules for appropriate behavior.

Canadian psychologist Virginia Douglas, known for her many contributions to our understanding of ADHD, was among the first to suggest that cognitive strategies might be used to help impulsive, hyperactive children gain control over their own behavior. In her laboratory at McGill University, Dr. Douglas observed ADHD children and concluded that hyperactivity was not the fundamental cause of their difficulties. Instead, she found that their problems stemmed from their poor impulse control and their inability to sustain attention. She described this succinctly as the inability to "stop, look, and listen" and explained, "These youngsters are apparently unable to keep their own impulses under control in order to cope with situations in which care, concentration, or organized planning are required."[13] Instead of taking the time to look over a problem carefully and consider alternative solutions, she added, they tend to jump in, acting on the first idea which occurs to them.

Dr. Douglas also speculated that ADHD children might be helped by teaching them better problem-solving strategies. The idea of providing ADHD children with "skills instead of pills" was received with enthusiasm, and beginning in the early 1970s, a number of cognitive training programs were designed to teach these skills.

These programs emphasize teaching the ADHD child to approach a task or a problem analytically by asking himself such questions as "What is my problem?" and "What is it I have to do?" As a second step, the child is instructed to think ahead and develop a plan by asking himself "How can I do this?" To prevent impulsive actions, the child might be encouraged to come up with alternative plans for solving the problem or completing the task, then to evaluate the relative merits of each plan and select the best one. These programs also teach children to evaluate their own performance while working on the task and to check frequently to be sure they are following their plan by asking "How am I doing?" and "Am I following my plan?" Because ADHD children often make careless errors, cognitive training programs also stress carefully checking work and correcting any errors. Finally, children are taught to praise themselves for successfully completing a task or solving a problem. Usually, too, they receive external rewards such as points or tokens for good performance.

After initial training on such tasks as puzzles and mazes, children are then taught to apply their new skills to schoolwork and social situations. For example, to help children learn to cope with difficult social situations in a less impulsive manner, training programs include role playing, training in social problem-solving skills, and exercises designed to teach cooperation with others.[14] In the home setting, cognitive self-control training has been used to teach ADHD children how to think through and resolve problems such as difficulty finishing homework and trouble getting ready to leave in the morning. In the classroom, cognitive training has been used to help children control their behavior, abide by the rules, and remain on-task with their work.[15]

In the United States and Canada, researchers have developed and tested several cognitive training programs, some of them quite elaborate and rather expensive. At the University of Illinois at Chicago, for example, one-hour training sessions were held twice weekly for three months, while a program at Columbia University provided two hours of weekly training for four months. If these services were provided by a therapist in private practice, parents could expect to pay anywhere from $1,000 to $2,000 or even more. When we factor in the demands made on parents and children in terms of time, along with the cost in actual dollars, we see that cognitive self-control training is not cheap. Is it worth it?

*The Evidence*

On the face of it, cognitive self-control training, in all its various guises, would certainly seem to be a promising approach to the problems of the ADHD child. It is a logical, well-thought-out approach which is consistent with what psychologists know about human behavior in general. More specifically, this approach is also solidly based on a very large body of research concerning the problems of children with ADHD.

Unlike other controversial treatments for children with learning and attention problems, cognitive training approaches have been studied in well-controlled experiments using sophisticated measurement techniques and statistical procedures. The scientific literature on the subject is so large as to be quite confusing. What does it show?

Early studies of the effectiveness of cognitive self-control techniques as treatment for children's learning and behavior problems were quite promising. In fact, as we discussed in Chapter 5, there is a small but convincing body of research which indicates that learning to use cognitive strategies can help children with learning problems improve their spelling, reading, and arithmetic skills. It can also help them memorize facts more efficiently and perform better on tests.

When we move from these circumscribed skills to the more complex arena of the behavior of the ADHD child at home, in school, and in other social settings, however, the results are disappointing. Although early studies reported improvements, these studies used children who were not considered to have ADHD. When researchers attempted to extend the approach to children who had actually been diagnosed with ADHD, results were much less impressive. Some studies using anger-control techniques have yielded promising results, but overall support for cognitive self-control strategies as a treatment for the more general problems of children with ADHD is quite limited.

Programs reporting some success have been those in which parents and other caregivers are taught to use the techniques in everyday settings and to combine them with reinforcement for appropriate behavior. When these other components are included, however, we cannot be certain which components are actually responsible for any improvements we observe. It may be the case that programs which combine cognitive self-control training with reinforcement for appropriate behavior are actually no more effective than reinforcement programs alone.

*Conclusions*

Cognitive training has not lived up to its early promise. In spite of the enormous appeal of this approach, results with ADHD children are generally modest. Used alone, cognitive self-control methods are clearly not as effective as stimulant medication or traditional behavior modification programs. In combination with these treatments, cognitive training may yield some additional benefits, but the amount of benefit obtained must be weighed against the cost. At best, cognitive training, like our other methods for treating ADHD, should be considered a management technique, not a cure. Parents who choose to employ this approach should be prepared to do so over a long period of time.

**SENSORY INTEGRATIVE THERAPY**

The approach to treating learning disabilities and ADHD known as sensory integrative therapy was developed by the late Dr. Jean Ayres, an occupational therapist who practiced in California. Her theory and treatment program have been described in numerous books and articles, and her approach is widely used by occupational therapists.

Dr. Ayres used the term "sensory integration" to refer to the brain's ability to organize and make use of incoming information from the various senses, such as vision, hearing, smell, taste, touch, motion, and temperature. To illustrate sensory integration, she used the example of peeling and eating an orange: the orange is sensed through the eyes, nose, and mouth and through the hands and fingers as they work together to coordinate peeling the orange and conveying it to the mouth. Sensations also come back to the brain from the teeth as they chew, the muscles in the tongue and throat as they convey the orange to the stomach, and so on. Thus, as she explained, "Sensory integration 'puts it all together.' "[16]

Like Dr. Harold Levinson (see Chapter 6), Dr. Ayres believed that the vestibular system[#] plays a critical role in learning disabilities and attention disorders. She viewed the vestibular system as the unifying system of the brain and stated that when it does not function properly, incoming sensory information is interpreted inconsistently and inaccurately. Problems which result include the following:

- ADHD. According to Dr. Ayres, "Much of the hyperactivity in children today is due to poor sensory integration." These children are easily distracted because the confusion in their brains makes it impossible for them to concentrate, and they "jump all over the classroom" because their brains are running out of control.

- Learning disabilities. Dr. Ayres believed that many learning problems are the result of poor sensory integration and that most learning-disabled children have some degree of sensory integrative dysfunction. In this regard, she linked learning disabilities with perceptual problems, sensory-motor deficits, and faulty eye movements.

- Speech and language disorders. While she acknowledged that not all speech and language problems are associated with vestibular dysfunction, Dr. Ayres stated that many children with these problems do evidence vestibular dysfunction and respond to sensory integrative therapy.

- Coordination problems. Difficulty with motor planning ("developmental dyspraxia") is considered one of the most common manifestations of sensory integrative dysfunction.

- Behavioral and social problems. According to Dr. Ayres, children with sensory integrative dysfunction are apt to be fussy, overly sensitive, and easily overwhelmed. They are also likely to have problems with social relationships.

In addition to the problems noted above, Dr. Ayres believed that many children with sensory integrative dysfunction also evidence *tactile defensiveness*; that is, they tend to react negatively and emotionally to a variety of touch sensations which would not bother most other people. Such a child is particularly sensitive about his face and head, so he usually finds it upsetting to have his face washed, his teeth cleaned, or his hair cut.

Since tactile defensiveness is an important manifestation of sensory integrative dysfunction, Dr. Ayres included tests to detect it as part of her assessment battery, known as the Southern California Sensory Integration Tests. Another important component of assessment is the test for *nystagmus*. Postrotary nystagmus is a series of rapid, reflexive, back-and-forth eye movements which occur after the body has been spun or rotated. According to Dr. Ayres, if the duration of nystagmus is too short, this indicates that the vestibular system is understimulated or is not processing input correctly. She believed that at least 50 percent of children with learning or language problems have too short a duration of nystagmus.

According to Dr. Ayres, between 5 and 10 percent of the children in this country have problems with sensory integration. Concerning the cause, she mentioned heredity, environmental toxins, and damage in utero or at birth, but added, "We know less about what causes sensory integrative dysfunction than we know what to do about it."

The "what-to-do-about-it" she proposed is sensory integrative therapy (SIT). Therapy consists of exercises which encourage the child to use as many nerve-cell connections as possible. Dr. Ayres believed that this would help him learn how to organize his brain, which, in turn, would make him better able to learn a broad variety of skills, including those of reading and writing.

Sensory integrative therapists believe that the average child does not need special experiences to help him develop these skills, because play provides him with the sensory stimulation and feedback needed for development. For the child with a sensory integrative dysfunction, however, special experiences are needed to help him organize his brain. These include brushing and rubbing of the skin, for example, to send tactile impulses to many regions of the brain. Deep-pressure exercises, vibration, and stretching exercises are used for the same reason. To stimulate the vestibular system, SIT incorporates activities like riding a scooter board down a ramp, and riding a bolster swing is used to help posture and balance.

*The Evidence*

The method developed by Dr. Ayres is widely used today. Its popularity can be explained in part by the fact that an exercise program seems like a "natural" way to treat a broad range of children's learning and behavior problems. (Indeed, Dr. Ayres herself extolled her approach as "completely natural.") Dr. Ayres's description of the problems of ADHD and learning-disabled children also accords with the fact that many of these youngsters are poorly coordinated and have social as well as behavioral problems.

But when we ask whether Dr. Ayres's theory is also consistent with what is currently known about the causes of ADHD and learning disabilities, we find significant discrepancies on several points:

- As we discussed in Chapter 6, there is no reason to believe that the vestibular system is primarily involved in regulating attention.

- Similarly, there is no support for the notion that the vestibular system is involved in speech and language disorders.

- Finally, the notion that reading disorders stem from faulty eye movements or problems with visual perception has been examined and found wanting, as we noted in Chapter 2.

Serious questions have also been raised about the tests Dr. Ayres used to assess vestibular dysfunction. Despite her claim that learning-disabled children and normal learners obtain very different scores on these tests, other researchers have *not* found these differences. In one study, for example, in which improved measures of vestibular function were used, tests of nystagmus did not indicate differences between learning-disabled and non-learning-disabled children. This researcher concluded that "there was no support for either the notion that vestibular function is related to academic performance or the vestibular dysfunction hypothesis among learning-disabled children."[17]

In another study, conducted by Dr. Robert Cummins at Victoria College in Australia, there were no differences between learning-disabled and non-learning-disabled children in measures of tactile defensiveness or in any of the measures used to assess sensory integrative dysfunction.[18] This, he concluded, throws doubt on both the diagnostic and the treatment procedures which are derived from Dr. Ayres's theory.

When we turn to research on the effectiveness of sensory integrative therapy as a treatment for ADHD and learning disabilities, we also find a lack of supporting evidence. In the twenty years since Dr. Ayres described her approach, many reports on SIT have been published, but few have met even the most minimal scientific standards. In fact, when Dr. William Feldman reviewed these reports for his 1990 book, *Learning Disabilities: A Review of Available Treatments*,[19] he could not find a single study which met truly rigorous standards of acceptability.

Since Dr. Feldman's survey of the literature, researchers in New Zealand and Toronto have conducted well-controlled studies of SIT, but their results do *not* support this approach. In New Zealand, Julie Densem and her colleagues compared SIT with a physical education program and found no effects of SIT on perceptual-motor skills, language development, self-concept, or handwriting skills. In both groups, children who were already reading made additional progress in reading, but this was not the case for children who were not already reading when the study began.[20]

At the University of Toronto, Dr. Tom Humphries and his associates compared SIT with a perceptual-motor training program. At the end of this expensive and time-consuming program (three sessions per week, for a total of seventy-two one-hour sessions), children in both groups showed some improvement in motor skills, but there was absolutely no improvement in visual perception, handwriting readiness, copying ability, self-concept, or cognitive, academic, language, or attentional skills.[21]

*Conclusions*

At this time, there is no consistent evidence from well-controlled studies that supports sensory integrative training as a treatment for children with learning or behavior problems. We do not know of any dangers associated with sensory integrative training. What we also do not know, however, is the extent to which children who are treated with this approach might benefit if other, proven treatment methods were used instead. Obviously, we cannot answer this question, nor can we recommend sensory integrative training for children with ADHD or learning disabilities.

**OPTOMETRIC VISION TRAINING**

The myth that learning disabilities are caused by visual problems was examined in Chapter 2. As we observed, there is an obvious connection between the eyes and the ability to read, but as far as reading delays and disabilities are concerned, current research overwhelmingly supports language deficiencies as the source of the difficulty. Nevertheless, this presumed connection between visual function and reading ability is a myth that simply refuses to die.

The notion that visual problems underlie learning problems lives on in part because it has been fostered by a group of optometrists[%] who offer a subspecialty known as "behavioral optometry" (sometimes called "developmental optometry"). According to behavioral optometrists, even if a child has perfect eyesight, he might still have difficulty interpreting and understanding what he sees. Behavioral optometrists argue that just as children progress from creeping to crawling to walking, there is a similar process which takes place in the development of visual skills. Since visual skills build one upon another, if a child somehow misses a step in the process, he won't have a solid foundation for all of the following steps. Even when this foundation has been solidly established, there are youngsters who develop problems when they enter school because they can't cope with spending long periods of time on tasks which require eye coordination before these skills are solidly in place.

Following their theory, behavioral optometrists have developed visual training programs which, they claim, will help the eyes function more efficiently and will enhance the child's ability to learn. The specific skills which they target in vision training programs include:

- Tracking: the ability of the eyes to follow a moving object smoothly and accurately.

- Fixation: the ability to locate and inspect a series of objects, one after the other, quickly and accurately.

- Binocularity: the ability of both eyes to work together smoothly and accurately.

- Focus change: the ability to make rapid changes from near to far objects, and vice versa.

Behavioral optometrists also think that poor eye-hand coordination and problems in visual perception contribute to learning disorders. They believe that training and practice in using the eyes and hands together will improve a child's ability to make discriminations of size, shape, location of objects, and so on. These skills, they state, are essential for academic progress.

What do behavioral optometrists suggest in the way of treatment? Their treatment programs, as actually employed, are extremely varied. In addition to eye exercises and the use of corrective lenses, many programs also include perceptual training exercises. Some programs include educational remediation and tutoring, while others incorporate adjunctive procedures such as biofeedback, nutritional counseling, and even family therapy. In fact, in one widely cited study,[22] a total of fifty-two different procedures were administered as part of the treatment program!

What kinds of children can be expected to benefit from vision therapy? In this area, the claims made by behavioral optometrists are almost as broad in scope as the treatment programs they use. Virtually all behavioral optometrists claim that their therapy will improve academic performance in children with learning problems. Some also claim that children who undergo training will show gains in intelligence test scores. Claims have also been made that vision therapy can enhance creativity;[23] that athletes who undergo vision therapy frequently report improved performance in their sport;[24] and that children with conditions as diverse as cerebral palsy, autism, and juvenile delinquency can benefit from vision therapy.

*The Evidence*

Can these sweeping claims for optometric vision therapy be substantiated? Before we consider the evidence, let us first look at whether research supports the behavioral optometrists' theory about the deficits they believe cause learning problems. Optometric training, in all its many guises, is based on the assumption that faulty eye movements and visual perceptual problems cause reading difficulties.

Are there really differences in eye-movement patterns between dyslexics and competent readers? Although a number of researchers have reported these differences, others have found the eye-movement patterns of dyslexics to be abnormal only in reading tasks, but not in nonreading visual tasks.[25] This, they believe, reflects the difficulty poor readers have when processing language.

Further, since the same patterns can be reproduced in competent readers simply by increasing the complexity of the material, it is likely that differences in eye movements do indeed *reflect* reading problems—they do not cause them.

If this is the case, there is no reason to believe that correcting eye-movement patterns would have any effect on reading. This is, in fact, what the evidence indicates, according to the results of a painstaking study conducted by Dr. Joel Fagan and his associates at the University of Calgary.[26] Using anti-motion-sickness medication instead of vision training, Dr. Fagan did find improved visual fixational stability in a group of dyslexic children. However, there was *no* relationship between improvement in eye movement and improvement in reading.

What about the assumption that visual-perceptual deficits cause learning disabilities? As we noted in Chapter 2, many learning-disabled children do have problems with visual perception and visual-motor coordination. In fact, much of the early work with learning-disabled children focused on correcting these problems on the assumption that improvements in learning would follow. Some of these programs, such as the well-known Frostig Program, involve training in discriminating various patterns, forms, and sounds. Others focus on physical exercises and balance training. From the limited research which has been done to evaluate this approach, we must conclude that it does *not* appear to be a useful treatment for learning disabilities.[27]

It is clear, then, that there is no evidence which supports the underlying assumptions of optometric vision training. Similarly, when we examine studies in which these methods have been applied, we find no evidence that they help learning-disabled children. In one study already mentioned, for example, poor readers received forty hours of training consisting of fifty-two procedures.[28] Although this study has been widely cited in support of vision training, the lack of an appropriate control group is only one of many flaws which make it impossible to conclude that vision training is effective in remedying learning disabilities.

*Conclusions*

In 1984, the American Academy of Pediatrics, in conjunction with the American Association for Pediatric Ophthalmology and Strabismus and the American Academy of Ophthalmology, issued a policy statement which included these conclusions:

> There is no peripheral eye defect that produces dyslexia and associated learning disabilities. Eye defects do not cause reversal of letters, words, or numbers... . [N]o known scientific evidence supports the claims for improving the academic abilities of dyslexic or learning-disabled children with treatment based on visual training, including muscle exercises, ocular pursuit or tracking exercises, or glasses (with or without bifocals or prisms).[29]

No one has voiced concern that any kind of eye damage might result from optometric vision training. However, as the American Academy of Pediatrics aptly pointed out, "Such training may result in a false sense of security which may delay or prevent proper instruction or remediation." They also cautioned that "the expense of such procedures is unwarranted."

We agree with the conclusions reached by this group and echo their concerns. At this time, it appears that optometric visual training is "less than meets the eye" and should not be used in the treatment of learning-disabled children.

\* Since there have been reports of higher levels of muscle tension in ADHD children, some researchers have actually used EMG feedback to treat children with learning and attention problems. Some have claimed positive results with this approach, but the studies are generally flawed and it is not clear how long after treatment the effects last or, indeed, whether the effects are any better than would be obtained with simple relaxation procedures alone.

# As we explained in Chapter 6, the vestibular system consists of the organs of balance in the inner ear. Within this system, one type of receptor is specialized for processing information about the forces of gravity, while a second type of receptor responds to the position and movement of the head.

% The public often confuses the terms "optometrist," "optician," and "ophthalmologist." *Opticians* are trained to make and fit corrective lenses, as prescribed by an optometrist or an ophthalmologist. *Optometrists* complete a four-year program in a college of optometry, where they are trained to examine the eyes, test visual acuity, and prescribe corrective lenses for visual problems. Because they are not physicians, optometrists cannot prescribe drugs or perform surgery. *Ophthalmologists* are physicians who, after completing their medical degrees, obtain three years or more of specialty training in diseases and disorders of the eyes.

# Chapter 9

## Miscellaneous Approaches

**NEURAL ORGANIZATION TECHNIQUE:**
**THE CHIROPRACTIC APPROACH**

The word "chiropractic" comes from the Greek words *cheir* and *prakikis* and means "done by hand." It is a theory of healing which is based on the belief that many illnesses are caused by mechanical disorders and deviations in the musculoskeletal system. Treatment usually involves physical manipulations ("corrective structural adjustments"), most commonly involving the spine and the arms and legs. Adjunctive methods used in chiropractic include physiotherapy procedures such as ultrasound, traction, and heat therapy. Since chiropractic is concerned with "the total person," nutritional counseling is often included as part of the treatment program.

Drs. Carl Ferreri and Richard Wainwright, both practicing chiropractors, have developed a chiropractic approach to treating learning disabilities which they call the Neural Organization Technique (NOT).[1] According to their theory, learning disabilities are caused by the misalignment of two specific bones in the skull, the sphenoid bone at the base of the skull and the temporal bones on the sides of the skull. This misalignment, they say, creates unequal pressure on different areas of the brain and causes the brain to malfunction.

Since the eye muscles are attached to the skull, if the cranial bones are not in the proper position, malfunctions in eye movement, known as "ocular lock," result. This condition, in turn, results in reading problems.

According to Ferreri and Wainwright, pelvic reflexes called "cloacal reflexes" are also a part of the overall problem. In a manner reminiscent of a line in the old song, "The knee bone's connected to the thigh bone," these reflexes influence many other reflexes throughout the body. If these reflexes are not synchronized, the chemical and mechanical functioning of the body will be impaired.

The treatment proposed by Ferreri and Wainwright consists of "spinal adjustments," specific body manipulations which they claim will correct misaligned cranial bones, faulty eye movements, and desynchronized pelvic reflexes. After these "adjustments" have been made, the individual is considered cured but must still undergo remedial tutoring to catch up academically.

What kinds of claims are made for this unorthodox approach to treating learning disabilities? We are told that after as few as one to eight sessions, learning and behavior symptoms improve dramatically or disappear, although follow-up visits are necessary to maintain improvement. We are told, too, about children who responded to treatment with improved emotional stability and reduced irritability, as well as improvements in hyperactivity, impulsivity, and behavior problems. Other children have reportedly responded with improvements in athletic ability and coordination, as well as dramatically improved school performance. We are even told that this form of treatment is 20 to 40 percent more effective than medication for ADHD.[2,3]

*The Evidence*

Chiropractic is a popular alternative health-care approach, and it is estimated that there are close to fifty thousand licensed practitioners in this country at the present time. However, there is no scientific evidence which supports the assumptions on which this approach is based, nor are there any well-controlled outcome studies of the effectiveness of chiropractic for any type of illness.

The theory underlying NOT is imaginative, but it is certainly not consistent with what is known about the cause of learning and attention problems. It is also not consistent with what is known about human anatomy, since standard medical textbooks state that the cranial bones do not move. In fact, since learning and behavior disorders are not listed by the American Chiropractic Association as being within the scope of practice of chiropractic, it appears that it is not even consistent with chiropractic theory.[4]

What about scientific evidence? Although studies have been cited by proponents of this approach, they have all appeared in obscure publications which do not require peer review. None of these studies have employed appropriate double-blind procedures, and in fact, all are so badly flawed that they can be considered little more than anecdotal evidence. In cases in which improvement is reported to have occurred as a result of treatment, it is impossible to rule out placebo effects or the effects of tutoring as causative factors.

*Conclusions*

In all respects, the chiropractic approach to treating learning disabilities and attention deficits is far outside the mainstream of current thought and clinical practice. It would appear to have no place in the treatment of children with ADHD or learning disabilities.

**IRLEN LENSES**

California psychologist Helen Irlen believes that learning disabilities and attention disorders are caused by a neurological condition she calls "Scotopic Sensitivity Syndrome" (SSS). This condition causes perceptual problems related to light source, light intensity, wavelength, and color contrast.[5]

Ms. Irlen states that due to their perceptual problems, individuals with SSS see the printed page differently from the way others see it. They may, for example, complain that letters seem to move on the page, or that words merge together, or that the print appears blurred or blotchy. Because they must use more energy and effort to read, people with SSS suffer discomfort, become fatigued, and have difficulty sustaining their attention over time. In addition to reading problems, people with SSS also report sensitivity to light, eyestrain, difficulty focusing, and other vision-related complaints.

According to Ms. Irlen, approximately 50 percent of reading-disabled individuals actually suffer from SSS. She claims that the great majority of them can be successfully treated with specially tinted lenses known as "Irlen lenses" or "Irlen filters." Although she cannot describe exactly how colored filters help individuals with SSS, she speculates that the filters selectively reduce specific troublesome wavelengths of light.

Since Ms. Irlen's appearance on the television program "60 Minutes" in 1988, her approach has attracted considerable attention. Public interest has been undoubtedly heightened by a number of glowing testimonials from people treated with this approach.

*The Evidence*

In Scotopic Sensitivity Syndrome, Helen Irlen claims to have identified a previously unrecognized visual-perceptual problem, which results in impaired reading ability. Ophthalmologists and optometrists, however, are not at all convinced that this is really the case. Instead, they argue that the "symptoms" of SSS are nothing more than ordinary vision problems which have not been properly diagnosed. Thus, problems such as headaches and eyestrain associated with reading, squinting, blinking, and rubbing the eyes might simply indicate that the sufferer needs glasses of the kind prescribed by any optometrist or ophthalmologist.

Ms. Irlen's notions concerning vision-related problems as a major cause of reading disorders is also not consistent with what is known about the underlying cause of most reading problems. As we have noted repeatedly, current research strongly suggests that most reading problems are language-based in origin.

In support of her theory, Ms. Irlen cites a study conducted in 1987 which reported improvements in academic performance in a group of students using the Irlen program.[6] In this study, however, tinted lenses were only one of *ten* interventions, which included the elimination of fluorescent lights and the use of colored paper, colored overlays, a tape recorder, and a magnifying bar. Students in this program were also provided with a tutor or reader and were given nontimed tests and oral or essay exams instead of true-false or multiple-choice tests. They were also permitted to prepare projects in place of written reports.

Dr. Russell Worrall, an optometrist on the National Council Against Health Fraud, reviewed this study and compared it to a primitive tribal remedy consisting of a sacred dance, a sacrificial lamb, a special tea, and numerous incantations. He concluded that, like the sacrificial lamb in the tribal remedy, the effectiveness of tinted lenses in this study remains very much open to question.[7]

Since this study appeared, several other investigators have evaluated the effectiveness of the Irlen lenses in improving reading. Sadly, most of these studies have never been published and so have never been subjected to critical analysis by peer reviewers. Many, such as the one described above, contain serious methodological flaws which prevent us from drawing conclusions about the contribution made by the lenses to the final outcome. In two studies in which proper controls were employed, results completely failed to support the effectiveness of the Irlen lenses in improving reading ability.[8,9]

*Conclusions*

Despite enthusiastic testimonials from patients who have been treated with Irlen lenses, there is no scientifically reproducible or consistent evidence that the lenses actually produce anything more than a placebo effect. There is also the danger that the use of Irlen lenses will result in some children with treatable visual problems going without appropriate treatment.

At this time, the Irlen lenses have no place in the treatment of learning disabilities. If your child appears to be bothered by vision-related complaints, he should receive a thorough eye examination from an optometrist or an ophthalmologist.

**OSTEOPATHIC TREATMENT**

Osteopathy is a system of diagnosis and treatment based on the belief that problems with the musculoskeletal system can adversely affect the functions of other systems in the body. Thus, it is assumed that human ailments generally result from such things as the pressure of displaced bones on nerves and are curable by physical manipulation.

Unlike a chiropractor, however, a doctor of osteopathy is a fully licensed physician who is qualified to prescribe medication and to practice all branches of medicine and surgery. In addition to standard medical training, osteopathic physicians receive training in examining patients through touch in order to diagnose illness and abnormalities. They are also trained to use osteopathic manipulative therapy (OMT), which includes thrusting techniques and rhythmic stretching and pressure. The objective of these techniques is to restore unrestricted motility to all parts of the body and to promote proper transmission of nerve impulses and circulation of blood, spinal fluid, and other bodily fluids.

According to osteopathic theory, skull malformations and dysfunctions in parts of the framework of the body can result from myriad sources, including genetic defects, birth injuries, toxins, and illness or injury after birth. In turn, these dysfunctions lead to abnormalities in neurological development and result in such problems as mental retardation, epilepsy, emotional disturbance, learning disabilities, and attention disorders.

Recently, some osteopathic physicians have proposed that children with learning and attention problems can benefit from OMT. According to their theory, OMT can help these children by correcting poor nervous system conduction and transmission of nerve impulses through correcting malfunctions in the musculoskeletal system.

*The Evidence*

Advocates of this approach are correct in claiming that children with learning and attention problems have documented problems in central nervous system functioning. However, we know of no consistent or compelling evidence linking these problems to malfunctions in the musculoskeletal system. Rather, the most current research indicates that the problems have their origin in neurotransmitter abnormalities within the central nervous system itself.[10]

In a recent study of the effects of OMT on the neurological development of children, weekly OMT treatments were given for six to twelve weeks to a group of youngsters with problems in a variety of areas, including learning, behavior, neuromotor functioning, and developmental delay.[11] The researchers concluded that OMT resulted in significant gains in sensory and motor performance in these children. However, there was no placebo control group in this study, the drop-out rate was very high, and the children studied constituted a poorly defined group. Thus, we cannot conclude that OMT is helpful to youngsters with learning and attention problems.

*Conclusions*

This treatment approach is not consistent with what is currently known about the causes of learning disabilities and attention problems, nor is there supporting evidence from scientific studies. Therefore, this treatment should not be employed with learning-disabled or ADHD children at this time.

## Concluding Remarks: Where Do We Go from Here?

Our society, like all other societies, has established a set of standards for its children. We expect them to attain certain levels of performance and achievement in the areas of development, behavior, and—increasingly important in this technological age—education. Unfortunately, not all children can meet these standards: despite their best efforts, those with learning and attention problems frequently fall short, disappointing themselves and those around them.

No child chooses to fail. Like the rest of us, children hunger for acceptance, approval, and recognition from others. As Dr. Melvin Levine, a pediatrician widely known for his work in the field of learning disabilities, writes:

> From the moment school-age children emerge from the bed covers each day until their safe return to that security, they are preoccupied with the avoidance of humiliation at all cost. They have a constant need to look good, to sidestep embarrassment, and to gain respect, especially from their peers.[1]

When a child consistently fails to meet the expectations of his parents, his teachers, and his peers, the effects can be devastating to the child's self-esteem. Repeated failure and frequent negative feedback can lead to profound feelings of helplessness ("I can't control my behavior"), worthlessness ("I'm bad" or "I'm stupid"), and despair ("What's the use of trying, since I'll never succeed?").

Witnessing the struggles and the pain of a youngster with learning or attention problems is agonizing to a parent. Parents of these youngsters, desperate to help their children but confused about the nature of the problem and the kinds of treatment most likely to help, may welcome any new treatment which offers hope. In the spirit of "How-can-it-hurt-to-try?," parents might be tempted to throw caution to the wind and expend time, money, and energy on unproven treatments, thereby placing a strain on limited family resources without obtaining any real benefit.

We hope that this book will prove a useful tool to parents and professionals as they strive to understand the difficulties faced by children with learning and attention problems, and to make informed choices about the best course of action to pursue. We hope, too, that the information contained in this book will help dispel the myths and misunderstandings about these conditions so that more children can receive the support and help they need to realize their potential.

It is now widely recognized that a significant number of children in our society experience learning disabilities and/or attention problems. We are encouraged by the amount of research devoted to the problems of these children and we are optimistic that, as our knowledge of the brain grows, so will our understanding of these disorders and our ability to treat them.

In the interim, parents and professionals must shoulder the responsibility for meeting the special needs of these children and advocating to see that their needs are recognized and met in the community. This is an enormous responsibility that requires a major investment of time, effort, caring, and commitment. To these people, and to the researchers who doggedly pursue knowledge to help our children, we extend two thumbs up and a heartfelt "Right on!"

With our best wishes,

Barbara Ingersoll
Sam Goldstein

Share this Book with your Friends!

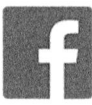    

# References

**CHAPTER 1: WHAT IS ATTENTION DEFICIT HYPERACTIVITY DISORDER?**

1. American Psychiatric Association, *Diagnostic and Statistical Manual of Mental Disorders*, 3rd. ed., rev. (Washington, D.C.: American Psychiatric Association, 1987).

2. P. Szatmari, D. R. Offord, and M. H. Boyle, "Ontario Child Health Study: Prevalence of Attention Deficit Disorder with Hyperactivity," *Journal of Child Psychology and Psychiatry* 30 (1989): 219-30.

3. R. A. Barkley, *Attention Deficit Hyperactivity Disorder: A Handbook for Diagnosis and Treatment* (New York: Guilford Press, 1990), 77.

4. J. H. Beitchman et al., "Prevalence of Psychiatric Disorders in Children with Speech and Language Disorders." *Journal of the American Academy of Child and Adolescent Psychiatry* 25 (1986): 528-35.

5. D. Cantwell and L. Baker, *Developmental Speech and Language Disorders* (New York: Guilford Press, 1987).

6. J. Biederman, J. Newcorn, and S. Sprich, "Comorbidity of Attention Deficit Hyperactivity Disorder with Conduct, Depressive, Anxiety and Other Disorders," *American Journal of Psychiatry* 148 (1991): 564-77.

7. Ibid.

8. R. A. Barkley, op. cit.

9. L. Smith, *Improving Your Child's Behavior Chemistry* (New York: Prentice Hall, 1976).

10. L. Smith, *Feed Your Kids Right* (New York: McGraw-Hill, 1979).

11. J. Rapp, *Is This Your Child? Discovering and Treating Unrecognized Allergies* (New York: William Morrow, 1991).

12. H. C. Lou, L. Henriksen, and P. Bruhn, "Focal Cerebral Hypoperfusion in Children with Dysphasia and/or Attention Deficit Disorder," *Archives of Neurology* 41 (1984): 825-29.

13. A. J. Zametkin et al., "Cerebral Glucose Metabolism in Adults with Hyperactivity of Childhood Onset," *New England Journal of Medicine* 323 (1990): 1361-66.

14. J. Kagan et al., "Information Processing in the Child: Significance of Analytic and Reflective Attitudes," *Psychological Monographs* 78 (1, Whole No. 578).

15. M. Gordon and B. B. Mettelman, *Technical Guide to the Gordon Diagnostic System* (Syracuse, N.Y.: Gordon Systems, 1987).

16. L. M. Greenberg, *Test of Variables of Attention Computer Program Manual* (St. Paul, Minn.: Attention Technology, 1990).

## CHAPTER 2: WHAT ARE LEARNING DISABILITIES?

1. J. M. Healy, *Endangered Minds: Why Children Don't Think and What We Can Do About It* (New York: Simon and Schuster, 1990).

2. J. F. Kavanagh and T. J. Truss, eds., *Learning Disabilities: Proceedings of the National Conference* (Parkton, Md.: York Press, 1988).

3. S. L. Smith, *No Easy Answers: The Learning Disabled Child at Home and at School* (Cambridge, Mass.: Winthrop Publishers, 1979).

4. J. H. Bruns, *They Can but They Don't: Helping Students Overcome Work Inhibition* (New York: Viking, 1992).

5. B. F. Pennington, *Diagnosing Learning Disorders: A Neuropsychological Framework* (New York: Guilford Press, 1991), 59.

6. M. Snowling and C. Hulme, "Speech Processing and Learning to Spell," in W. Ellis, ed., *All Language and the Creation of Literacy* (Baltimore, Md.: Orton Dyslexia Society, 1991).

7. J. W. Gilger, B. F. Pennington, and J. C. DeFries, "A Twin Study of the Etiology of Comorbidity: Attention Deficit Hyperactivity Disorder and Dyslexia, *"Journal of the American Academy of Child and Adolescent Psychiatry* 31 (1992): 343-48.

8. K. J. Rowe and K. S. Rowe, "The Relationship Between Inattentiveness in the Classroom and Reading Achievement (Part B): An Explanatory Study," *Journal of the American Academy of Child and Adolescent Psychiatry* 31 (1992): 357-68.

9. J. C. DeFries et al., "Colorado Reading Project: An Update," in D. Duane and D. Gray, eds., *The Reading Brain: The Biological Basis of Dyslexia* (Parkton, Md.: York Press, 1991).

10. C. Wright-Strawderman and B. L. Watson, "The Prevalence of Depressive Symptoms in Children with Learning Disabilities," *Journal of Learning Disabilities* 25 (1992): 258-64.

11. A. Mehrabian and S. R. Ferris, "Inference of Attitudes from Nonverbal Communication in Two Channels," *Journal of Consulting Psychology* 31 (1967): 248.

12. B. P. Rourke, *Nonverbal Learning Disabilities: The Syndrome and the Model* (New York: Guilford Press, 1989).

13. S. D. Smith et al., "Specific Reading Disability: Identification of an Inherited Form Through Linkage and Analysis," *Science* 219 (1983): 1345-47.

14. DeFries et al., "Colorado Reading Project."

15. N. A. Badian, "Reading Disability in an Epidemiological Context: Incidence and Environmental Correlates," *Journal of Learning Disabilities* 17 (1984): 129-36.

16. A. M. Galaburda, "Anatomy of Dyslexia: Argument Against Phrenology," in D. D. Duane and D. B. Gray, eds., *The Reading Brain: The Biological Basis of Dyslexia* (Parkton, Md.: York Press, 1991).

17. G. W. Hynd et al., "Brain Morphology in Developmental Dyslexia and Attention Deficit Disorder/Hyperactivity," *Archives of Neurology* 47 (1990): 919-26.

18. Pennington, *Diagnosing Learning Disorders*, 115.

19. S. Weintraub and M. M. Mesulam, "Developmental Learning Disabilities of the Right Hemisphere," *Archives of Neurology* 40 (1983): 463-68.

20. R. W. Woodcock, *Woodcock-Johnson Psychoeducational Battery —Revised* (Allen, Tex.: Teaching Resources, 1989).

21. L. M. Dunn and F. C. Markwardt, *Peabody Individual Achievement Test* (Circle Pines, Minn.: American Guidance Service, 1970).

22. D. Wechsler, *Wechsler Intelligence Scale for Children—III* (New York: Psychological Corporation, 1991).

## CHAPTER 3: HOW NEW TREATMENTS ARE EVALUATED: SCIENCE, PSEUDOSCIENCE, AND QUACKERY

1. B. Russell, *History of Western Philosophy* (New York: Simon and Schuster, 1945).

2. F. Franks, *Polywater* (Cambridge, Mass.: MIT Press, 1981).

3. S. Wolf, "Effects of Suggestion and Conditioning on the Action of Chemical Agents in Human Subjects," *Journal of Clinical Investigation* 29 (1950): 100.

4. H. K. Beecher, *Measurement of Subjective Responses: Quantitative Effects of Drugs* (New York: Oxford University Press, 1959).

## CHAPTER 4: EFFECTIVE TREATMENTS FOR ADHD

1. R. A. Barkley, "A Review of Stimulant Drug Research with Hyperactive Children," *Journal of Child Psychology and Psychiatry* 18 (1977): 137-65.

2. S. Goldstein, *Managing Attention Disorders in Children* (New York: Wiley, 1990).

3. F. R. Sallee, R. L. Stiller, and J. M. Perel, "Pharmacodynamics of Pemoline in Attention Deficit Disorder with Hyperactivity," *Journal of the American Academy of Child and Adolescent*

*Psychiatry* 31 (1992): 244-51.

4. C. K. Conners and K. C. Well, *Hyperkinetic Children: A Neuropsychosocial Approach* (Beverly Hills, Calif.: Sage Publications, 1986), 97.

5. J. Rapoport, "Medical News. Stimulant Therapy for Attention Disorders," *Journal of the American Medical Association* 248 (1982): 279-87.

6. R. A. Barkley, "Placebo 'Side Effects' and Ritalin," *Clinical Child Psychology Newsletter* 3 (1989): 2.

7. "The Cult of Greed and Power," *Time,* May 6, 1991.

8. R. A. Barkley, "Predicting the Response of Hyperkinetic Children to Stimulant Drugs: A Review *Journal of Abnormal Child Psychology* 4 (1976): 327-48.

9. H. C. Parker et al., "Medical Management of Children with Attention Deficit Disorders: Commonly Asked Questions," *CH.A.D.D.ER* 5 (1991): 17-19.

10. R. Klorman et al., "Clinical Effects of a Controlled Trial of Methylphenidate on Adolescents with Attention Deficit Disorder," *Journal of the American Academy of Child and Adolescent Psychiatry* 29 (1990): 702-9.

11. K. D. Gadow, E. E. Nolan, and J. Sverd, "Methylphenidate in Hyperactive Boys with Comorbid Tic Disorder: II. Short- Term Behavioral Effects in School Settings," *Journal of the American Academy of Child and Adolescent Psychiatry* 31 (3) (1992): 462-71.

12. R. Hunt, S. Lau, and J. Ryu, "Alternative Therapies for ADHD," in L. Greenhill and B. Osman, eds., *Ritalin: Theory and Patient Management* (New York: Mary Ann Liebert, 1991).

13. M. K. Dulcan, "The Safe and Effective Use of Psychotropic Medications in Adolescents and Children: Information for Parents and Youth on Psychotropic Medications," *Journal of Child and Adolescent Psychopharmacology* 2 (2) (1992): 91.

14. T. W. Phelan, *1-2-3: Magic! Training Your Preschoolers and Preteens to Do What You Want* (Glen Ellyn, Ill.: Child Management, 1984).

15. R. A. Barkley, *Attention Deficit Hyperactivity Disorder: A Handbook for Diagnosis and Treatment* (New York: Guilford Press, 1990).

16. S. Goldstein and M. Goldstein, *Managing Attention Disorders in Children: A Guide for Practitioners* (New York: John Wiley and Sons, 1990).

17. M. Rapport, A. Murphy, and J. S. Bailey, "The Effects of a Response Cost Treatment Tactic on Hyperactive Children," *Journal of School Psychology* 18 (1990): 98.

18. E. D. Heins, J. W. Lloyd, and D. P. Hallahan, "Cued and Non-Cued Self-Recording of Attention to Task," *Behavior Modification* 10 (1986): 235-54.

19. H. Parker, *Listen, Look, and Think: A Self-Regulation Program for Children* (Plantation, Fla.: ADD Warehouse, 1991).

20. S. S. Zentall, The Education of ADHD Youth: An Earthquake in Colors," *CH.A.D.D.ER* 5 (1991): 8.

21. R. R. Davila, M. L. Williams, and J. T. MacDonald, *Memorandum from the United States Department of Education* (Washington, D.C.: Office of Special Education and Rehabilitative Services, September 16, 1991).

## CHAPTER 5: EFFECTIVE TREATMENTS FOR LEARNING DISABILITIES

1. D. J. Johnson, "Review of Research on Specific Reading, Writing, and Mathematics Disorder," in J. F. Kavanagh and T. J. Truiss, eds., *Learning Disabilities: Proceedings of the National Conference* (Parkton, Md.: York Press, 1988).

2. W. Feldman, *Learning Disabilities: A Review of Available Treatments* (Springfield, Ill.: Charles C. Thomas, 1990).

3. W. E. Pelham et al., "The Dose-Response Effects of Methylphenidate on Classroom Academic and Social Behavior in Children with Attention Deficit Disorder," *Archives of General Psychiatry* 42 (1985): 948-52.

4. R. S. Stephens, W. E. Pelham, and R. Skinner, State-Dependent and Main Effects of Methylphenidate and Pemoline on Paired-Associate Learning and Spelling in Hyperactive Children," *Journal of Consulting and Clinical Psychology* 52 (1984): 104-13.

5. E. Richardson et al., "Effects of Methylphenidate Dosage in Hyperactive Reading-Disabled Children: II. Reading Achievement," *Journal of the American Academy of Child and Adolescent Psychiatry* 27 (1988): 78-87.

6. R. A. Barkley, G. J. DuPaul, and M. B. McMurray, "Attention Deficit Disorder with and without Hyperactivity: Clinical Response to Three Doses of Methylphenidate," *Pediatrics*, in press.

7. Richardson et al., "Effects of Methylphenidate Dosage."

8. R. Gittelman, D. F. Klein, and I. Feingold, "Children with Reading Disorders: II. Effects of Methylphenidate in Combination with Reading Remediation," *Journal of Child Psychology and Psychiatry* 24 (1983): 222-33.

9. A. W. Alexander et al., "Phonological Awareness Training and Remediation of Analytic Decoding Deficits in a Group of Severe Dyslexics," *Annals of Dyslexia* 41 (1991): 193-206.

10. R. Gittelman and I. Feingold, "Children with Reading Disorders: I. Efficacy of Reading Remediation," *Journal of Child Psychology and Psychiatry* 24 (1983): 167-91.

11. I. S. Brown and R. H. Felton, "Effects of Instruction on Beginning Reading Skills in Children at Risk for Reading Disability," *Reading and Writing* 2 (1990): 223-41.

12. P. Lindamood, Personal Communication, 10/10/92. Additional information available from Lindamood-Bell Learning Processes, 416 Higuera, San Luis Obispo, Calif. 94301.

13. T. E. Scruggs et al., "Mnemonic Facilitation of Learning Disabled Students' Memory for Expository

Prose," *Journal of Educational Psychology* 79 (1987): 27-34.

14. C. A. Kearney and R. S. Drabman, "The Write-Say Method for Improving Spelling Accuracy in Children with Learning Disabilities," *Journal of Learning Disabilities* 26 (1993): 52-56.

15. T. W. Lombardo and R. S. Drabman, "Teaching LD Children Multiplication Tables," *Academic Therapy* 20 (1985): 437-42.

16. T. E. Scruggs and D. Tolfa, "Improving the Test-Taking Skills of Learning-Disabled Students," *Perceptual and Motor Skills* 60 (1985): 847-50.

17. R. T. Brown and N. Alford, "Ameliorating Attentional Deficits and Concomitant Academic Deficiencies in Learning Disabled Children Through Cognitive Training," *Journal of Learning Disabilities* 17 (1984): 20-26.

18. D. H. Schunk and P. D. Cox, "Strategy Training and Attributional Feedback with Learning Disabled Students," *Journal of Educational Psychology* 78 (1986): 201-9.

19. H. E. Pigott, J. W. Fantuzzo, and P. W. Clement, "The Effects of Reciprocal Peer Tutoring and Group Contingencies on the Academic Performance of Elementary School Children," *Journal of Applied Behavior Analysis* 19 (1986): 93-98.

20. K. M. Jones, J. K. Torgeson, and M. A. Sexton, "Using Computer Guided Practice to Increase Decoding Fluency in Learning Disabled Children: A Study Using the Hint and Hunt I Program," *Journal of Learning Disabilities* 20 (1987): 122-28.

21. R. K. Olson and B. W. Wise, "Reading on the Computer with Orthographic and Speech Feedback," *Reading and Writing* 4 (1992): 107-44.

## CHAPTER 6: PILLS AND POTIONS

1. L. Pauling, "Orthomolecular Psychiatry," *Science* 160 (1968): 265-71.

2. A. Hoffer et al., "Treatment of Schizophrenia with Nicotinic Acid and Nicotinamide," *Journal of Clinical and Experimental Psychopathology* 18 (1957): 131-58.

3. A. Cott, "Orthomolecular Approach to the Treatment of Learning Disabilities," *Schizophrenia* 3 (1971): 95-105.

4. M. Colgan and L. Colgan, "Do Nutrient Supplements and Dietary Changes Affect Learning and Emotional Reactions of Children with Learning Difficulties? A Controlled Series of 16 Cases," *Nutrition and Health* 3 (1984): 69-77.

5. A. Brenner, "The Effect of Megadoses of Selected B-Complex Vitamins on Children with Hyperkinesis: Controlled Studies with Long-Term Follow-Up, "*Journal of Learning Disabilities* 15 (1982): 258-64.

6. R. F. Harrell et al., "Can Nutritional Supplements Help Mentally Retarded Children? An Exploratory Study," *Proceedings of the National Academy of Science* 78 (1981): 574.

7. L. E. Arnold et al., "Megavitamins for Minimal Brain Dysfunction," *Journal of the American Medical Association* 240 (1978): 2642-43.

8. J. Kershner and W. Hawke, "Megavitamins and Learning Disorders: A Controlled Double-Blind Experiment," *Journal of Nutrition* 109 (1979): 819-26.

9. R. H. Haslam, J. T. Dalby, and A. W. Rademaker, "Effects of Megavitamins on Children with Attention Deficit Disorders," *Pediatrics* 74 (1984): 103-11.

10. *Megavitamin and Orthomolecular Therapy in Psychiatry: Task Force Report No. 7*. (Washington, D.C.: American Psychiatric Association, 1973).

11. H. N. Levinson, *Total Concentration: How to Understand Attention Deficit Disorders, with Treatment Guidelines for You and Your Doctor* (New York: M. Evans, 1990).

12. Ibid.

13. T. W. Uhde et al., "Historical and Modern Concepts of Anxiety: A Focus on Adrenergic Function," in J. C. Ballenger, ed., *Biology of Agoraphobia* (Washington, D.C.: American Psychiatric Press, Inc., 1984).

14. S. P. Wise and J. L. Rapoport, "Obsessive-Compulsive Disorders: Is It Basal Ganglia Dysfunction?" in J. L. Rapoport, ed., *Obsessive-Compulsive Disorder in Children and Adolescents* (Washington, D.C.: American Psychiatric Press, Inc., 1989).

15. H. N. Levinson, "Dramatic and Favorable Responses of Children with Learning Disabilities or Dyslexia and Attention Deficit Disorder to Antimotion Sickness Medications: Four Case Reports," *Perceptual and Motor Skills* 73 (1991): 723-38.

16. J. E. Fagan et al., "The Failure of Antimotion Sickness Medication to Improve Reading in Developmental Dyslexia: Results of a Randomized Trial," *Developmental and Behavioral Pediatrics* 9 (1988): 359-66.

17. W. G. Crook, *The Yeast Connection: A Medical Breakthrough* (Jackson, Tenn.: Professional Books, 1986).

18. W. G. Crook, *Help for the Hyperactive Child* (Jackson, Tenn.: Professional Books, 1991).

19. Executive Committee of the American Academy of Allergy and Immunology, "Candidiasis Hypersensitivity Syndrome," *Journal of Allergy and Clinical Immunology* 78 (1986): 271-73.

20. W. E. Dismukes et al., "A Randomized, Double-Blind Trial of Nystatin Therapy for the Candidiasis Hypersensitivity Syndrome," *New England Journal of Medicine* 323 (1990): 1717-23.

21. L. Galland and D. Buchman, *Superimmunity for Kids* (New York: E. P. Dutton, 1988).

22. E. A. Mitchell et al., "Clinical Characteristics and Serum Essential Fatty Acid Levels in Hyperactive Children," *Clinical Pediatrics* 26 (1987): 406-11.

23. I. Colquhoun and S. Bunday, "A Lack of Essential Fatty Acids as a Possible Cause of Hyperactivity

in Children," *Medical Hypotheses* 7 (1981): 673-79.

24. M. G. Aman, E. A. Mitchell, and S. H. Turbott, "The Effects of Essential Fatty Acid Supplementation by Efamol in Hyperactive Children," *Journal of Abnormal Child Psychology* 15 (1987): 75-90.

25. L. E. Arnold et al., "Gamma-Linoleic Acid for Attention-Deficit Hyperactivity Disorder: Placebo-Controlled Comparison to D-Amphetamine," *Biological Psychiatry* 25 (1989): 222-28.

26. D. R. Wood, F. W. Reimherr, and P. H. Wender, "Treatment of Attention Deficit Disorder with dl-Phenylalanine," *Psychiatry Research* 16 (1985): 21-26.

27. E. D. Nemzer et al., "Amino Acid Supplementation as Therapy for Attention Deficit Disorder," *Journal of the American Academy of Child and Adolescent Psychiatry* 25 (1986): 509-13.

28. A. J. Zametkin et al., "Treatment of Hyperactive Children with d-Phenylalanine," *American Journal of Psychiatry* 144 (1987): 792-93.

29. C. R. Wilsher et al., "Piracetam and Dyslexia: Effects on Reading Tests," *Journal of Clinical Psychopharmacology* 7 (1987): 230-37.

30. P. T. Ackerman et al., "A Trial of Piracetam in Two Subgroups of Students with Dyslexia Enrolled in Summer Tutoring," *Journal of Learning Disabilities* 24 (1991): 542-49.

## CHAPTER 7: DIETARY INTERVENTIONS

1. D. J. Rapp, *Is This Your Child? Discovering and Treating Unrecognized Allergies* (New York: William Morrow, 1991).

2. C. K. Conners, *Feeding the Brain: How Foods Affect Children* (New York: Plenum Press, 1989).

3. B. Feingold, *Why Your Child Is Hyperactive* (New York: Random House, 1974).

4. National Institutes of Health, "Defined Diets and Childhood Hyperactivity: Consensus Conference," reprinted in *Journal of the American Medical Association* 248 (1982): 290-92.

5. E. H. Wender, "The Food Additive-Free Diet in the Treatment of Behavior Disorders: A Review," *Developmental and Behavioral Pediatrics* 7 (1986): 35-42.

6. B. Weiss et al, "Behavioral Responses to Artificial Food Colors, *Science* 207 (1980): 1487-89.

7. K. S. Rowe, "Synthetic Food Colourings and 'Hyperactivity': A Double-Blind Crossover Study," *Australian Pediatric Journal* 24 (1988): 143-47.

8. Rapp, *Is This Your Child,* 34.

9. Ibid., 351.

10. Ibid., 329.

11. Ibid., 354.

12. Ibid., 40.

13. "American Academy of Allergy and Immunology: Position Statements: Controversial Techniques, "*Journal of Allergy and Clinical Immunology* 67 (1981): 333-38.

14. Rapp, op. cit., 503.

15. J. Egger et al., "Controlled Trial of Oligoantigenic Treatment in the Hyperkinetic Syndrome," *The Lancet*, March 9, 1985, 540-45.

16. B. J. Kaplan et al., "Dietary Replacement in Preschool-Aged Hyperactive Boys," *Pediatrics* 83 (1989): 7-17.

17. F. C. Bennett and R. Sherman, "Management of Childhood 'Hyperactivity' by Primary Care Physicians, "*Journal of Developmental and Behavioral Pediatrics 4* (1983): 88-93.

18. R. J. Prinz, W. A. Roberts, and E. Hantman, "Dietary Correlates of Hyperactive Behavior in Children," *Journal of Consulting and Clinical Psychology* 48 (1980): 760-69.

19. M. L. Wolraich et al., "Dietary Characteristic of Hyperactive and Control Boys and Their Behavioral Correlates," *Journal of the American Dietetic Association* 86 (1986): 500-4.

20. D. Behar et al., "Sugar Challenge Testing with Children Considered Behaviorally 'sugar reactive,' " *Journal of Nutrition and Behavior* 1 (1984): 277-88.

21. E. H. Wender and M. V. Solanto, "Effects of Sugar on Aggressive and Inattentive Behavior in Children with Attention Deficit Disorder with Hyperactivity and Normal Children," *Pediatrics* 88 (1991): 960-66.

22. M. Gross, "Effect of Sucrose on Hyperkinetic Children," *Pediatrics* 74 (1984):876-78.

23. R. Milich and W. E. Pelham, "The Effects of Sugar Ingestion on the Classroom and Playgroup Behavior of Attention Deficit Disordered Boys," *Journal of Consulting and Clinical Psychology* 54 (1986): 714-18.

24. C. K. Conners, *Feeding the Brain: How Foods Affect Children* (New York: Plenum Press, 1989).

25. N. Rosenthal, *Seasons of the Mind* (New York: Bantum, 1990).

## CHAPTER 8: TRAINING APPROACHES TO TREATMENT

1. *Woman's Day,* September 3, 1991, 102-6.

2. *Reader's Digest,* May 1992, 105-8.

3. J. F. Lubar and M. N. Shouse, "EEG and Behavioral Changes in a Hyperkinetic Child Concurrent with Training of the Sensorimotor Rhythm (SMR): A Preliminary Report," *Biofeedback and Self-*

*Regulation* 1 (1976): 293-301.

4. J. M. Halperin et al., "Relationship Between Stimulant Effect, Electroencephalogram, and Clinical Neurological Findings in Hyperactive Children," *Journal of the American Academy of Child Psychiatry* 25 (1986): 820-25.

5. J. H. Satterfield et al., "Topographic Study of Auditory Event-Related Potentials in Normal Boys and Boys with Attention Deficit Disorder with Hyperactivity," *Psychophysiology* 25 (1988): 591-606.

6. C. A. Mann et al., "Quantitative Analysis of EEG in Boys with Attention Deficit Hyperactivity Disorder: Controlled Study with Clinical Implications," *Pediatric Neurology* 8 (1992): 30-36.

7. NeuroAuto Therapy Institute, *Brainwave Biofeedback Training for Attention Deficit Disorder* (Louisville, Ky.: NeuroAuto Therapy Institute).

8. M. A. Tansey, "Brainwave Signatures: An Index Reflective of the Brain's Functional Neuroanatomy," *International Journal of Psychophysiology* 3 (1985): 89-99.

9. D. Kade, "Biofeedback to Neurotherapy," *PADDA-DATA, Newsletter of the Peninsula Attention Deficit Disorder Association,* (1992): 8-14.

10. B. Brandell, Letter/Advertisement (Wood Dale, Ill.: Autogenics, 1992).

11. A. R. Luria, *The Role of Speech and the Regulation of Normal and Abnormal Behaviors* (New York: Liveright, 1961).

12. L. Vygotsky, *Thought and Language* (New York: John Wiley and Sons, 1962).

13. V. I. Douglas, "Are Drugs Enough? To Treat or Train the Hyperactive Child," in R. Gittelman-Klein, ed., *Recent Advances in Child Psychopharmacology,* (New York: Human Sciences Press, 1975), 203.

14. S. P. Hinshaw, B. Henker, and C. K. Whalen, "Self-Control in Hyperactive Boys in Anger-Inducing Situations: Effects of Cognitive-Behavioral Training and of Methylphenidate," *Journal of Abnormal Child Psychology* 12 (1984): 55-77.

15. R. A. Barkley, A. P. Copeland, and C. Sivage, "A Self-Control Classroom for Hyperactive Children," *Journal of Autism and Developmental Disorders* 10 (1980): 75-89.

16. A. J. Ayres, *Sensory Integration and the Child* (Los Angeles: Western Psychological Services, 1979), 5.

17. H. J. Polatajko, "A Critical Look at Vestibular Dysfunction in Learning-Disabled Children," *Developmental Medicine and Child Neurology* 27 (1985): 283-92.

18. R. A. Cummins, "Sensory Integration and Learning Disabilities: Ayres' Factor Analyses Reappraised," *Journal of Learning Disabilities* 24 (1991): 160-68.

19. W. Feldman, *Learning Disabilities: A Review of Available Treatments* (Springfield, 111.: Charles C.

Thomas, 1990).

20. J. F. Densem et al., "Effectiveness of a Sensory Integrative Therapy Program for Children with Perceptual-Motor Deficits," *Journal of Learning Disabilities* 22 (1989): 221-29.

21. T. Humphries et al., "A Comparison of the Effectiveness of Sensory Integrative Therapy and Perceptual-Motor Training in Treating Children with Learning Disabilities," *Developmental and Behavioral Pediatrics* 13 (1992): 31-40.

22. D. J. Getz, "Learning Enhancement Through Visual Training," *Academic Therapy* 15 (1980): 457-66.

23. Optometric Extension Program Foundation, *What Is Visual Training?* (pamphlet) (Santa Ana, Calif.: OEP, 1984).

24. Ibid.

25. K. Rayner, "Eye Movements and the Perceptual Span: Evidence for Dyslexic Typology," in G. T. Pavlidis and D. F. Fisher, eds., *Dyslexia: Its Neuropsychology and Treatment* (New York: Wiley, 1986).

26. J. E. Fagan et al., "The Failure of Antimotion Sickness Medication to Improve Reading in Developmental Dyslexia: Results of a Randomized Trial," *Developmental and Behavioral Pediatrics* 9 (1988): 359-66.

27. K. Kavale and P. D. Mattson, " 'One Jumped Off the Balance Beam': Meta-Analysis of Perceptual-Motor Training," *Journal of Learning Disabilities* 16 (1983), 165.

28. Getz, "Learning Enhancement Through Visual Training."

29. Committee on Children with Disabilities, American Academy of Pediatrics, "Learning Disabilities, Dyslexia, and Vision," *Pediatrics* 74 (1984): 150-51.

## CHAPTER 9: MISCELLANEOUS APPROACHES

1. C. A. Ferreri and R. B. Wainwright, *Breakthrough for Dyslexia and Learning Disabilities* (Pompano Beach, Fla.: Exposition Press of Florida, 1984).

2. E. V. Walton, "Chiropractic Effectiveness with Emotional, Learning and Behavioral Impairments," *International Review of Chiropractic* 29 (1975): 2-5, 21-22.

3. J. M. Giesen, D. B. Center, and R. A. Leach, "An Evaluation of Chiropractic Manipulation as a Treatment of Hyperactivity in Children," *Journal of Manipulative and Physiological Therapeutics* 12 (1989): 353-63.

4. American Chiropractic Association, *Chiropractic: State of the Art, 1991-1992* (Arlington, Va.: American Chiropractic Association, 1991).

5. H. Irlen, *Reading by the Colors: Overcoming Dyslexia and Other Reading Disabilities Through the Irlen*

*Method* (Garden City Park, N.Y.: Avery Publishing Group, 1991).

6. L. Adler and M. Atwood, "Poor Readers, What Do They Really See on the Page? A Study of a Major Cause of Dyslexia (West Covina, Calif.: East San Gabriel Regional Occupational Program, 1987). Cited in R. S. Worrall, "Detecting Health Fraud in the Field of Learning Disabilities," *Journal of Learning Disabilities* 23 (1990): 207-12.

7. Worrall, "Detecting Health Fraud."

8. SPELD (S.A.), "Tinted Lenses and Dyslexics: A Controlled Study," *Australian and New Zealand Journal of Ophthalmology* 17 (1989): 137-41.

9. P. Blaskey et al., "The Effectiveness of Irlen Filters for Improving Reading Performance: A Pilot Study," *Journal of Learning Disabilities* 23 (1990): 604-12.

10. R. D. Hunt et al., "Neurobiological Theories of ADHD and Ritalin," in L. Greenhill and B. Osman, eds., *Ritalin: Theory and Patient Management* (New York: Mary Ann Liebert, Inc., 1991).

11. V. M. Frymann, R. E. Carney, and P. Springall, "Effect of Osteopathic Medical Management on Neurologic Development in Children," *Journal of the American Osteopathic Association* 92 (1992): 729-44.

## CONCLUDING REMARKS:
## WHERE DO WE GO FROM HERE?

1. M. D. Levine, *Developmental Variation and Learning Disorders* (Cambridge, Mass.: Educators Publishing Service, Inc., 1987).

# Addenda

**INFORMATION AND SUPPORT GROUPS FOR PARENTS**

**ADDA**

(Attention-Deficit Disorder Association)

4300 West Park Boulevard

Plano, TX 75093

> This nationally represented group is a consortium of local support groups for families of children with Attention Deficit Disorder. ADDA is an excellent referral source and well aware of the majority of support groups throughout the country.

**ADDAG**

(Attention Deficit Disorder Advocacy Group)

8091 South Ireland Way

Aurora, CO 80016

(303) 690-7548

> This parent association is very active in providing support to parents, professionals, and educators.

**ADDendum**

(Quarterly newsletter for adults who have Attention Deficit Disorder)

Box 296

Scarborough, NY 10510

**Association for Children and Adults with Learning Disabilities**

National Headquarters

4156 Library Road

Pittsburgh, PA 15234

(412) 341-1516

> This is a nonprofit national organization concerned with the education of children

with learning disabilities and attention disorders. It publishes a newsletter five times per year and has local and state chapters throughout the country.

**ATTENTION Please!**

(Bimonthly newsletter for children with ADD)

2106 Third Avenue North

Seattle, WA 98109-2304

**CH.A.D.D.®**

(Children and Adults with Attention Deficit Disorders)

499 NW 70th Avenue, #308

Plantation, FL 33317

(305) 587-3700

Comprised of well over four hundred chapters nationally and internationally, this organization is dedicated to providing support and information to parents and professionals. CH.A.D.D. is an excellent source for helping parents and adults with ADD identify local resources. The group publishes several manuals and brochures concerning parent advocacy and services available for handicapped children. CH.A.D.D. also publishes a newsletter ten times a year and organizes the largest national conference on ADD in the country.

**LEARNING DISABILITIES ASSOCIATION OF CANADA**

Alberta

145-11343 61st Avenue

Edmonton T6H 1M3

(403) 448-0360

British Columbia

203-15463 104th Avenue

Surrey V3R 1N9

(604) 588-6322

Manitoba

301-960 Portage Avenue

Winnipeg R3G 0R4

(204) 774-1821

New Brunswick
138 Neil Street
Fredericton E3A 2Z6
(506) 459-5521

Newfoundland
P.O. Box 8632, Station A
St. John's A1B 3T1
(709) 754-3665

Northwest Territories
P.O. Box 242
Yellowknife X1A 2N2
(403) 873-6378

Nova Scotia
55 Ochterloney Street
Dartmouth B2Y 1C3
(902) 464-9751

Ontario
124 Merton Street, 3rd Floor
Toronto M4S 2Z2
(416) 487-4106

Prince Edward Island
P.O. Box 1081
Charlottetown C1A 7M4
(904) 892-9664

Quebec (Aqeta)
300-284 rue Notre-Dame O
Montreal H2Y 1T7
(514) 847-1324

Saskatchewan

Albert Community Centre

26-610 Clarence Avenue S.

Saskatoon S7H 2E2

(306) 652-4114

Yukon Territory

P.O. Box 4853

Whitehorse Y1A 4N6

(403) 668-5167

**CH.A.D.D. Canada, Inc.**

P.O. Box 23007

Ottawa, Ontario K2A 4E2

(613) 591-3761

**RECOMMENDED TEXTS FOR PARENTS**

Bain, L. J. *Attention Deficit Disorders*. New York: Dell Publishing Company, 1986.

Fowler, M. C. *CH.A.D.D. Educator's Manual*. Fairfax, Va.: CH.A.D.D., 1992.

Fowler, M. C. *Maybe You Know My Kid: A Parents' Guide to Identifying, Understanding and Helping Your Child with Attention-Deficit Hyperactivity Disorder*. New York: Birch Lane Press, 1990.

Goldstein, S., and Goldstein, M. *Hyperactivity: Why Won't My Child Pay Attention*. New York: Wiley-Interscience Press, 1992.

Gordon, M. *ADHD/Hyperactivity: A Consumer's Guide*. DeWitt, N.Y.: GSI Publications, 1991.

Ingersoll, B. *Your Hyperactive Child: A Parent's Guide to Coping with Attention Deficit Disorder*. New York: Doubleday, 1988.

Levine, M. *Keeping A Head in School: Students Book About Learning Abilities and Learning Disorders*. Cambridge, Mass.: Educator's Publishing Service, 1990.

Osman, B. B. *Learning Disabilities: A Family Affair*. New York: Warner Books, 1979.

Parker, H. C. *The ADD Hyperactivity Handbook for Schools*. Plantation, Fla: Impact Publications, 1992.

Parker, H. C. *The ADD Hyperactivity Workbook for Parents, Teachers and Kids*. Plantation, Fla.: Impact Publications, 1990.

Silver, L. *The Misunderstood Child: A Guide for Parents of Learning Disabled Children.* New York: McGraw-Hill, 1984.

**RECOMMENDED VIDEOS FOR PARENTS**

Barkley, R. *ADHD—What Can We Do?* (video). New York: Guilford, 1992.

Barkley, R. *ADHD—What Do We Know?* (video). New York: Guilford, 1992.

Goldstein, S., and Goldstein, M. *Educating Inattentive Children* (video). Salt Lake City, Utah: Neurology Learning & Behavior Center, 1990.

Goldstein, S., and Goldstein, M. *It's Just Attention Disorder* (video and user's guide). Salt Lake City, Utah: Neurology Learning & Behavior Center, 1991.

Goldstein, S., and Goldstein, M. *Why Won't My Child Pay Attention?* (video). Salt Lake City, Utah: Neurology Learning & Behavior Center, 1989.

Phelan, T. *Attention Deficit Hyperactivity Disorder* (two-part video and book). Glen Ellyn, Ill.: Child Management, Inc. 1990.

www.ingramcontent.com/pod-product-compliance
Lightning Source LLC
Chambersburg PA
CBHW050216230526
45470CB00001B/409